DON'T PANIC, YOU ARE HAVING A BABY

Dr. Anthony Cohn

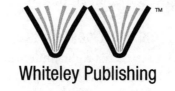

Whiteley Publishing

Photograph credit: Elny Cohn
Published by Whiteley Publishing Ltd
First soft cover edition 2013

ISBN 978-1-908586-58-2

CONTENTS

For The Whole Mishpocha

The Strict laws of the Sabbath, which includes avoiding lighting a flame, may be broken for the benefit of a lady in childbirth. If she asks for light, her neighbour may light a candle for her... The Master said.

Isn't that obvious, what we are really learning here is that even if the woman is blind we can still light a candle for her; You might have thought that as she cannot see, there is no benefit to her in having a light and it should be forbidden. However, it is important that we do this to alleviate her anxiety, because she will say, even if I can't see, I will be reassured to know that with the light, my friends will be able to see better and allow me to have a safer delivery.

Babylonian Talmud
Sabbath 128b
c.5ᵗʰ Century

ACKNOWLEDGEMENTS

Working at West Herts Hospital Trust – Watford and Hemel Hempstead Hospitals – has been for me a tremendous privilege. Much of this is due to the outstanding colleagues that I work with. I think that our unit is fantastic, and the relationships between team members on all levels exemplary. I am particularly grateful to my consultant colleagues who seem to tolerate my foibles and idiosyncrasies. Each of them could have produced a far better book than this. I thank them for their support and encouragement and look forward to many more years working together. I count my blessings that every day is a day that I want to come to work.

Spolf, Gav, Eitan and Elny (you know who you are) as ever you make everything and anything worthwhile. Emily and all at Whiteley Publishing, thank you for all your work and belief. Without you this book would not exist.

I have written this book in good faith. I have tried to be as up to date as possible. I have given an honest opinion but acknowledge that in medicine things are rarely black and white and different people can hold different views, so if this book does mislead or confuse you I apologise. Thank you for looking at this book. I hope that everything goes well for the future.

INTRODUCTION

There are hundreds of books out there about pregnancy and childbirth, so why bother writing another one? That is a very good question.

Essentially this book has grown out of answering questions about pregnancy and childbirth. Crucially, they are the type of questions that friends ask me because they know that I am a Paediatrician. So these are the answers that people want to know, but might not know who to ask.

I think the main question people want to know is: "How will this affect my baby?" Whether they are asking about medical conditions in pregnancy or the choices that you can make.

We will examine a lot of different parts of obstetric and postnatal care, but these will essentially be from the baby's perspective.

I hope that this book will be helpful and reassuring, as it is impossible to over emphasize the impact that parents have on their children. It is important for your children that you feel as good as you possibly can and this includes feeling good about yourself.

Getting it right - the first time

As anybody with children will tell you, there is only one correct way of dealing with childbirth and babies and that is, to do everything exactly as we have done it. By all means try something different; only don't blame us when it all goes terribly wrong.

We are so convinced about how right we are that we demand that other people should be given a choice, as long as they only choose what we want them to. Of course other people shouldn't be allowed to have any choice when they will choose the things that we disagree with.

Coming clean, I am a Paediatrician. I don't get any funding outside of medical practice so I have no particular axe to grind. I believe that achieving happy, confident and rested parents is more important to the well-being of a child than chasing after goals which may be impossible to attain. This means that I might appear controversial and may not be completely politically correct at all times. I will however try to give you more information than opinion, but still, please feel free to disagree with me.

In reality, children are very resilient and thankfully, despite all of our best intentions and efforts, as long as we do things with love they seem to thrive and flourish whatever it is that we actually do.

Motherhood

There is a by-product of conception, which is well known to every single mother, but is often not recognised by others. In fact, the moment that the sperm hits the egg and fertilises it, a substance is released which floods the mother's body and stays with her for the rest of her life. That substance is guilt. Anything bad that happens to the baby during its entire lifetime is always the mother's fault.

Somehow this guilt, like the most effective parasite in the world, gnaws away at your self-belief until you are so overwhelmed that you can't imagine that something is not your fault. The cynics amongst us say that this guilt is so overpowering that it also consumes all sanity and perspective that might have existed previously.

There are many ways that as a mother you can fail your baby. You may have failed to carry the pregnancy to term, you may have failed to push the baby out naturally and you have probably failed in some aspect of feeding or settling your baby.

This feeling does not get any better. Whether your child catches a cold or does not win the fancy dress competition it is likely that you will identify some thing that, if only you had done it a bit better, could have prevented this unimaginable tragedy.

By some fluke of nature, this rarely affects fathers. Instead, it seems that the fertilising sperm contained the very last drop of their sensitivity. So that, now relieved of this, they are able to say and do exactly the right thing to make their partners feel completely terrible.

So, I may not be a mother, but even if I don't know how you feel, I think I know a bit about what you feel. I hope that this book may make things a bit easier for you.

I could tell you that it's not your fault, but even if you pretended to agree with me I know that deep down you probably wouldn't believe me.

For interfering, unhelpful relatives:

∇ Remember, if you are struggling to find the wrong thing to say you can always rely on the 'are you sure...' question. After the parents have made a decision which they may have agonised over for some time, this question guarantees that you can sow the seeds of doubt.

∇ Unfortunately you may find that the new parents have difficulty expressing their gratitude towards you and may even appear hostile. Do not be deterred, this is merely a stage that they are going through and in no way allow this to diminish your input.

Parenting as a competitive sport - how to win without really playing

For a large number of people parenting is becoming increasingly competitive. Some people will boast of how long they continued to work for whilst pregnant, others about how long they rested. How much music did you play to your baby whilst in the womb? Did you give your baby the benefits of a normal labour/water birth/home birth? Did your baby get good Apgar scores? This is just the start of it.

The competition intensifies with events for the most stressed, most laidback, most exhausted, most well slept, most saintly, most blessed and so on: and for children - most trying, most angelic, most advanced, best eater, best grower, best and worst vomiter, sleeper and pooer. Many families enrol in as many categories as possible believing they are due some special achievement award. Part of the competition involves letting everybody else know how well you are doing compared to how badly they are doing. Broadly there are two groups, the blessed earth mother for whom everything is wonderful and amazing; the pinnacle of whose life is being covered in baby vomit. Alternatively there is the martyr, every problem she faces is just so much more than anybody else's and the only way she can bear her miserable lot is to share her burden with anybody that will listen.

Apart from the fact that most of these things are completely beyond anybody's control most of them really don't matter. If everybody is happy, well that's just wonderful. If you have the occasional bright moment; rejoice and if you are just about surviving, that might be as good as it gets for now. But it will get better.

Chances are you are probably too tired or busy to actually compete very well in any case. Also, remember that there is no way of checking your rival's claims so how do you know that they are not making it all up. This gives you a number of choices:

- Feel even more depressed and more of a failure.
- Listen attentively. Then bitch like crazy behind their backs.
- Agree not to talk about babies with them - unlikely to be successful for more than 12 seconds.
- Argue with them that they are actually missing the whole point of parenthood.
- Fabricate. Remember nobody is checking up on you either. So maybe your baby did sleep all night and you are looking ragged because you had 12 hours of unbridled passion. Or the doctor could have said that your baby's eating habits have been shown to reduce his chances of becoming obese in later life - and all that chocolate delivered at an early stage will teach his body to handle it so much better when he gets older. If you are very considerate you
- might tell them that you are only joking and if you are only slightly considerate you may only tell them when they have changed their whole lives around to be a bit more like yours.

Congratulations - you are going to be a parent. From now on nothing will go as planned

An important underlying principle of parenthood is finding out just how little control you actually have. This can be very scary for people who may be used to having quite a lot of control in their lives. From the time of conception you realise that you cannot determine very much. You may have an idealised plan of how you want your pregnancy to progress and how you want your baby baby to be born, but your pregnancy may not go to plan and your baby may need to be born in a completely different way.

Your baby may look different to the baby of your imagination and may have different ideas as to how to feed and sleep. Believe me, as they get older they do not behave more in tune with your wishes. The only reasonable advice is to 'go with the flow'. Learn to accept those things that you have no power over and don't spend so much time worrying about tomorrow that you forget to enjoy today.

A Paediatrician's view of OBSTETRICS

I hope that I am not getting carried away here and although I work closely with Obstetricians I only see the results of their and their patients' labours. From my point of view we want to try and make things as safe as possible for your baby and you. You can become a prime target for people wanting to sell you their own idea of how you should behave. You may feel pressurised into doing things or to stop doing things believing that this is essential for a successful outcome for you and your baby. It is important that you feel comfortable with the antenatal care plan that you choose, so it is worth taking a closer look and seeing what the advantages and drawbacks of antenatal care are.

What is safe antenatal care - disturbing the hornets' nest?

I probably need to get out some protective clothing before saying what comes next. Anyway, here goes. There seem to be two completely opposite schools of thought as regards pregnancy and delivery; their positions are so entrenched that to the outsider it seems as if they barely communicate. We might call these groups the 'harbingers of doom' or the 'eternal optimists'. This is a little less contentious than saying doctors and midwives. A famous maxim is that the Obstetrician sees complications where none exist whilst the midwife refuses to see complications even when they are staring him in the face.

What do the harbingers of doom say?

This group which is, if you like, the medical group, view pregnancy as a journey of high risk with disaster looming at every possible juncture. They believe that if anything can go wrong it almost certainly will. The best way to deal with this is to have lots of tests and investigations, to be monitored up to the eyeballs and have a high-tech delivery with thousands of doctors in attendance. If and only if everything is all right will you be allowed to see your baby.

What about the eternal optimists?

These people have a different approach. Pregnancy is a completely natural process, medicalising it deprives the mother of a wonderful experience. Any medical intervention is likely to cause irreparable damage to mother, child and family unit. Delivery can take place anywhere you wish. Monitoring of labour may be a necessary evil but should be kept to a minimum and once born you should immediately cuddle your baby. After this essential event is complete, we can have a look at your baby to see if he is OK.

So, who is right?

The simple answer is both of them and neither of them. Like a lot of things in medicine, obstetric care has become a victim of its own success. We no longer see childbirth as a time of great danger for mother and baby. Advances in care have slashed maternal and neonatal mortality to such a small number that you are unlikely to know anybody who has not had a successful outcome to their pregnancy.

For example, things have progressed so much that we tend to think of terrible labours as ones that are prolonged, painful or have ended with an instrumental delivery. Our grandmothers and great-grandmothers would have taken this in their stride and offered thanks for surviving childbirth and delivering a live baby.

There are other forces at play. A lot of people have a very negative attitude to modern medicine and doctors and think that the whole baby thing was going just fine until these 'Doctors,' who not surprisingly were all male, muscled in on it and tried to take things away from the good old birth attendant and midwife. Modern Male Medicine turned a beautiful natural event into an illness.

There is undoubtedly some truth in this. A 'hospital' pregnancy will involve more visits, more tests and an increased chance of having an instrumental delivery or a Caesarean section. A lot of these will take place 'just to be on the safe side' which, in other words, means that they are almost certainly not necessary. So, although the Caesarean section rate continues to rise, it doesn't seem to be making any impact on the outcome for babies.

Worryingly, because medical care is more expensive, the people that pay the bills (the government) seem to favour the 'it will all come up roses' approach. Because they calculate how much cheaper it would be if pregnancy did not have any health problems linked to it, they hope to save money and face by providing cheap care claiming that it is actually better.

The doom laden approach is not without its problems, not only may it increase anxiety and intervention, but also many people complain of a process that seems clinical, uncaring and impersonal as if you really are on a production line.

After all, childbirth has changed; we are having fewer children and are usually having children out of choice. We want to value and enjoy the pregnancy and feel that it is a period for growth in lots of areas - not just the physical. We want to be informed and to make choices. We want to have some ownership of our bodies.

In the vast majority of pregnancies, it doesn't matter what you do. They will progress easily without any problem and result in a lovely healthy baby. A very small minority of pregnancies will be problematic for the mother, the baby or both. Unfortunately, the only way to see if you are at risk is to do the tests.

Recently, although the number remains extremely low, there has been a slight increase in serious complications of pregnancy in the UK. It is quite possible that this is because we are downplaying the importance of medical care in pregnancy and failing to recognise warning signs.

Help, get me out of here!

I don't want to confuse or distress you. Here are some questions that you might want to ask your team:

- Am I healthy, or do I have a condition, which might cause some risk to my baby or me?
- Will I be checked for common problems of pregnancy such as high blood pressure or diabetes?
- How will the pregnancy be monitored? Are all the tests really necessary? Do I need more or less tests?
- Will the labour be adequately monitored?
- What facilities will you have if my baby or I get into difficulty during labour?

- If my baby is born needing help, will this be immediately available?

Once you are happy with all the answers and this might mean asking if the answer is good enough, then it doesn't really matter which approach you take.

Antenatal tests

In pregnancy you will be offered a whole variety of tests to check how well you and your baby are doing. It is important to appreciate that increasing medical care has revolutionised pregnancy and childbirth. Maternal mortality is about 1% of what it was 100 years ago and much of this is directly related to changes in medical care.

There are different reasons for doing these tests and it can be useful to know what they are for. Basically they can be divided into a few groups:

- Checking that you are healthy
- Checking that the pregnancy is not harming you; the mother
- Monitoring the wellbeing of the baby
- Identifying if the baby has any problems

Many conditions that could be dangerous tend to creep up suddenly, often by the time we know that they are there, significant damage has already been done. Because of this, it is a good idea to check a few things routinely during your pregnancy - especially your blood pressure and blood sugar or glucose.

High blood pressure can be dangerous for the mother and also harmful for the baby. If the mother has high blood pressure, the placenta may be affected so that the blood supply to the baby is reduced. A reduced blood supply means that your baby may not receive all of the oxygen and nutrients necessary to grow. In addition to poor growth, there are other changes, which will help your baby cope with the situation. For example in order to take as much oxygen as possible the baby will produce extra red blood cells. Although this sounds like a good idea, it means that the blood becomes thicker and will flow more slowly. Occasionally this in itself can cause problems. So, if your blood pressure is rising you can be offered treatment to try and prevent these complications.

Similarly if your glucose is high, this means that your baby will receive too much glucose. This can cause problems whilst still in the womb, as the baby can grow too much and get too big which can lead to a difficult delivery. After birth your baby could have problems maintaining their own glucose levels.

The reason for this is that if your glucose levels are high, your baby will be exposed to high glucose levels in the womb. To deal with this they will produce extra insulin - the hormone that helps glucose go into our cells, so reducing blood glucose. After delivery, the baby's glucose supply drops immediately the cord stops pulsating or is clamped. The baby's high insulin production will still continue with the risk that without extra sugar from outside, his own blood sugar levels will fall and this can be very dangerous. If your blood sugar levels are high you can be given advice and treatment to bring the levels back to normal. If they remain a problem, it is important that the team delivering your baby are aware so that they can provide your baby with feeds that prevent the baby's blood sugar falling.

Other tests may be useful. Knowing your blood group can be vital if you need a transfusion, but you will also have your 'rhesus' status checked as well. The reason for this is to check if you have, or might develop antibodies to your baby's blood. If this were to happen then the antibodies could cross the placenta and break down the baby's blood causing him to become anaemic. This is a rare but serious condition. You and your baby would need close monitoring. Sometimes babies need treatment in the womb, before delivery with a blood transfusion. Other babies with this problem will need close monitoring after they are born and are likely to be quite jaundiced and may also require blood transfusions. Without the blood tests it would be difficult to predict if this was likely to happen. If we know that this could happen then we can be prepared which means that treatment is likely to be better.

Some blood tests identify if you are carrying any infections that can be passed on to your baby and also whether you - and hence your baby - are protected against other infections such as rubella - German measles.

Very occasionally pregnancy can trigger more serious illness in a mother and, if this is suspected, further tests will need to be done. Sometimes the only 'cure' for the mother will be delivering the baby. This should always be done after discussions with all the doctors involved. As a general rule we would place the mother's health as the most important factor and taking this into account would want to plan a delivery that would give her baby every chance of doing well.

Ultrasound Scans

One of the most amazing advances of the last thirty years has been the widespread availability of ultrasound scans. The fact that we can see our children before they are born is amazing. Happily there do not seem to be any risks associated with ultrasound scans so you can have as many as you like without harming your baby. I am aware that there were some concerns about the safety of scanning but these seem to be completely without foundation.

It is interesting that doctors and prospective parents have a different view of an ultrasound scan. For most parents it is a time of excitement and the first chance to see your baby. Whilst that is wonderful of itself, the main medical reason for ultrasonography is to assess the well being of your baby and see if there are any problems that might need addressing.

In this respect scans can provide a lot of information. From a few weeks of age, a scan can show you whether or not you are pregnant. At 12 weeks or so it can be used to estimate the date of delivery of your baby and also to check that your baby does not have any major problems. At this stage the 'nuchal thickness' will be measured. This is the thickness of the tissues in the neck. This is increased in some medical abnormalities - including Down's syndrome.

If any abnormalities are detected then further investigations or scans can be necessary. Later scans can monitor the overall growth of your baby and check that they are receiving a good blood supply. The scans can look more closely at all of the organs to check that they are growing properly. Repeated scans are very important in multiple pregnancies to make sure that each baby is growing well.

This information can be of great value. Sometimes babies might need treatment whilst still in the womb - for example; blood transfusions. Without the information from the scan this would not be known and equally importantly the treatment would be carried out using the scanner to point out where to place the injection.

In other cases, scans can identify when a baby is struggling, for example by not growing as well as expected and inform the decision about allowing the pregnancy to continue or delivering your baby early. In other cases, a problem may have been identified which will need immediate treatment at birth. In this case the paediatric team can be primed to start treatment immediately rather than waiting for problems to arise. In some cases this will mean transferring your care to a place which has appropriate paediatric support.

Sometimes, the scans reveal changes which, whilst not immediately worrying, will need monitoring - such as some kidney abnormalities. If these are not known about in advance and managed early, they might cause long-term problems.

Every silver lining has a cloud and ultrasound scanning is not exempt from this. The two main issues relating to scanning would be that it could make you panic unnecessarily but also give you a false sense of security.

A lot of the changes that we see could actually be normal. We might pick something up in your baby and suggest that this is monitored regularly. This can make you think that there is something terribly wrong with your baby. However most of the time these changes amount to nothing and no treatment is ever necessary. We have just made you worry. Your 100 year old grandmother who has never been sick in her life may have the same 'abnormality' as your unborn baby - only your grandmother never had a scan in her life so has lived happily and healthily, completely oblivious to the 'potential problem'. It is surprising how many congenital abnormalities are first picked up at post-mortem in people over the age of 90!

The other thing to point out is that the scan is never 100% perfect and sometimes even quite significant abnormalities can be missed. The quality of scans is improving all the time but things can still slip through the net. That is why the person doing the scan will write 'NAD' rather than 'normal' on the report. This stands for Nothing Abnormal Detected. There are also some abnormalities, which will not be detectable by ultrasound.

Occasionally the scan will pick up problems, which are so severe that you will be faced with the heart wrenching decision about whether to continue with the pregnancy or not.

Excellent help is available via antenatal results and choices (ARC) www. arc-uk.org Helpline: 020 7631 0285

CHILDBIRTH - A BABY'S VIEW - THE GOOD NEWS FOR BABIES

As far as your baby is concerned, it doesn't really matter what happens, as long as he comes out safely.

Getting ready

Life outside the womb is very different to life inside. In order to cope with this, babies have an amazing ability to adapt rapidly to massive changes. Essentially, in the womb, all of the baby's oxygen is supplied through the placenta, via the mother's blood. Before birth babies have very low levels of oxygen in their blood. To make life a little easier they have special haemoglobin, which allows them to utilise this small amount of oxygen to maximum advantage.

It is easier to understand the circulation before birth - the foetal circulation - if we first look at the postnatal or 'adult' circulation.

After birth, we use our lungs to breathe. Blood flows through the lungs where it picks up oxygen and releases carbon dioxide. This blood then goes to the left side of the heart from where it is pumped through the arteries to the body to provide oxygen to all of the organs.

The organs and tissues of the body take out some of the oxygen and replace it with the waste product - carbon dioxide. This blood travels through the veins to the right side of the heart from where it is pumped into the lungs to start the cycle again.

Because unborn babies don't need their lungs to breathe, a number of things happen. Firstly, instead of all of the blood going through the lungs most blood actually 'bypasses' them. In order to achieve this, there is a hole - the foramen ovale - between the two sides of the heart so that blood entering into the right side, passes directly to the left side of the heart without going through the lungs. There is also a blood vessel - the ductus arteriosus - that joins the pulmonary artery - the main blood vessel leading to the lungs - with the aorta, the main artery supplying the body. This also works as a bypass route: blood that is heading to the lungs is diverted through this blood vessel to go directly to the body instead.

After birth it is important that these routes close, so that all the blood will flow through the lungs. This begins to happen at birth and takes a few days to complete.

The other challenge is to make the lungs ready for breathing. In the womb the lungs secrete a lot of fluid, which is important for lung growth. So, they are really overflowing with fluid during pregnancy and need to be 'empty' within a short time of delivery.

The one thing more stressful than having a baby is being born. During normal labour babies' adrenaline and stress hormones rise to phenomenal levels. As one of my teachers used to say "If you have been born; you have already lived through the most stressful event of your life!"

There is a positive aspect to this, as it helps to prepare the baby for life outside. Adrenaline makes the lungs resorb the liquid that they produce so that at delivery they can be filled with air and breathing can start. The preparation of the lungs for breathing takes place during labour rather than during delivery. So, as soon as the baby has gone through a normal delivery it's lungs will be 'empty' and waiting to be filled with air. This can be an important consideration if you are having a water birth - because if the baby breathes whilst underwater it is going to get a load of bathwater into its lungs, not an ideal start to life.

The other major thing that happens during labour is that, at times, the blood supply to the baby is effectively reduced or even cut off. This leads to even less oxygen being delivered to the tissues, a situation that is called hypoxia. This occurs particularly during contractions. The way that the baby deals with this is to prioritise where the blood is going to flow to, with the most important organs being the brain, heart and adrenal glands.

Another special adaptation of babies is that they hold stores of energy in their heart. So, if the heart is being deprived of oxygen, it has a large energy reserve to help keep it pumping.

If you think watching a baby being born is a miraculous sight, it's nothing when you think about what is going on inside the baby at the time.

Medicines in pregnancy and labour

Clearly it is best to avoid medicines in pregnancy whenever possible. Nobody can forget the Thalidomide tragedy when a drug that was thought to be safe had such devastating results.

However, nowadays any drug that is prescribed to a pregnant woman will have been rigorously tested. It is remarkable how safe most drugs seem. Certainly if there was even the slightest suspicion that a drug may be dangerous then your doctor would not prescribe it or your pharmacist dispense it - so it is important to let them know if you are pregnant - especially in the early stages.

Sometimes, not taking medication may be more of an issue than taking it. For instance, unborn babies are quite susceptible to fever. So if you have a high temperature it is probably better to take something to bring this down rather than leave it untreated.

If you have a medical condition, which needs treatment, then you really must take the medication. Often there is a choice of medicines to take, so we can try and find the one that is safest for your baby, but having a sick or ill mother is never in your baby's best interest.

Because some drugs cross the placenta they can impact on your baby. As I said, this rarely causes problems but if we know what drugs you are taking, we can deal with this until the drug is removed from your baby's body. For example if you are on blood pressure tablets your baby's blood pressure may be a bit low for the first few days of life. If you have had to have morphine for severe pain for a long period of time, your baby may have some withdrawal effects. These are not hard to treat but the more we know beforehand the easier it is to deal with.

It is highly unlikely that any of these drugs are going to have any long-term effects on your baby

The drugs that we would be concerned about would be recreational drugs - morphine/cocaine/amphetamines etc, alcohol and smoking which are much more likely to cause long-term harm.

During delivery you may receive painkillers, which can cross the placenta and make the baby a bit sleepy. Your baby may need a little help until the effects of these have worn off. Yet again they cause no long-term problems and this is not a reason to stop you having full pain relief in labour.

Monitoring and Foetal Distress

One of the most fantastic achievements of modern medicine has been to make childbirth essentially safe for mother and baby. Although the baby has a lot of ways of dealing with the stress of delivery sometimes it can be too much and this can lead to serious problems.

The challenge that Obstetricians and midwives face is trying to detect when a baby is becoming 'exhausted'. Once this stage is reached it becomes increasingly necessary to deliver the baby before things get worse in order to avoid damage to the baby. This would normally mean proceeding to an instrumental delivery or a Caesarean section. Finding the right balance is an impossible task and currently means that in most hospitals there is a rise in the number of assisted deliveries.

There are different ways of monitoring a baby's wellbeing during labour. The essential one is to listen to its heartbeat. This is either done electronically (using cardiotocography - a CTG) or by listening intermittently with a special stethoscope. Stress can cause the baby's heart to react in a number of different ways, with a slowing heart rate being the most ominous sign. If there are signs of the baby becoming distressed, then the obstetric team will act to speed up the delivery.

In some cases they may wish to check the baby's blood gas. This is a very useful guide to how much a baby may be struggling. If the baby is not getting enough oxygen and becoming distressed, acids will start building up in its blood and this can be checked by a simple blood test. Blood is taken from the babies scalp, using a very small specially designed blade. The results of this test are crucial to deciding how long it is safe to continue with labour.

These investigations do involve the baby. To measure his heart rate, a 'foetal scalp electrode' can be placed, through the birth canal onto the baby's head. This can cause a small bruise, but is not linked to any long-term problem. Similarly a blood test might cause a small scar, which will fade within a few days.

Babies can also respond to stress by passing meconium - baby poo. This can be detected because it stains the amniotic fluid. If a baby has passed meconium before being born, this alerts people to the fact that things are getting difficult. Occasionally, meconium can enter into the baby's lungs and cause significant breathing problems. A midwife or Paediatrician will want to attend to the baby immediately, to reduce the chances of this happening and to help the baby if needed.

WHAT DIFFERENCE DOES IT MAKE TO THE BABY?

Babies are remarkably resilient. They really don't seem to mind how they are delivered. Obviously our desired delivery is a simple normal labour with as little medical input as necessary. It doesn't always work like that; so let's look at some of the alternatives.

Pain relief and epidurals

There is a whole bizarre argument about pain relief in labour, remember it's labour not martyrdom. There is no evidence that pain is a vital part of labour. Being in agony during the delivery is not an essential component of good motherhood and the drugs used for pain relief will have no lasting impact on the baby.

My brother remembers attending antenatal classes when the subject of analgesia arose. Every father in the room discussed his disdain for drugs and mentioned how his partner would deliver their child with a mixture of breathing exercises and moral support. When it came to his turn he said, 'I don't much worry about myself, but I don't think that my wife should suffer for my principles and she should have everything she can to make her as comfortable as possible!'

However you choose to spend labour is going to make little difference in the long term to your baby. It is possible that having an epidural may prolong the pushing stage, as you may not have as much sensation as without one. It is possible that the chance of needing a little bit of help at the end, say with Ventouse or forceps, may be increased, but this is also not going to affect your baby in the long term. Epidurals can cause some side effects in mothers but these are usually of little significance and/or short lived.

Pain killing drugs, such as pethidine, can cross over into the baby, to make the baby a little sleepy as well. Normally this is no problem at all; occasionally the baby may need some extra stimulation or monitoring until the drug is passed out of his system. If this is necessary this will only be for a short time.

Instrumental delivery

The two types of instrumental delivery are forceps and vacuum extraction - Ventouse. These are used if the baby is nearly out, but needs to be delivered more quickly than he is being pushed out. They are ways of giving a helping hand to the final stages of delivery.

Forceps are specially designed to go around the baby's head. Once applied, the Obstetrician will pull the baby out gently. Forceps have been around for many hundreds of years and although the process sounds fairly gruesome, they are actually remarkably safe. Sometimes they can cause a little bit of bruising, which usually settles within a few days.

The Ventouse is a rubber cap, which is applied to the baby's head. A vacuum is created to help keep this on. The Obstetrician can then use this to pull the baby out. Quite often the cap can leave a little raised bruise, a chignon, which resolves in a few days.

Babies born by forceps and Ventouse often have quite a lot of moulding. This is when the head can appear a bit squashed. This is usually because the baby's head has been stuck for a time, before the Ventouse or forceps were applied.

Instrumental deliveries appear to be quite safe for babies. Obviously, the fact that they are needed in the first place suggest that the baby has been in difficulty and it has become necessary to speed up delivery. Any real risks are linked to why the forceps or Ventouse were needed in the first place and the forceps and Ventouse are used to reduce the overall risk to your baby.

Caesarean sections

There are lots of ways of describing Caesarean sections. Normally they are divided into elective sections, ones which are planned and emergency ones, which are unplanned.

The Obstetrician will also describe which part of the womb the baby was delivered through. This is normally the lower part or section of the womb. So, they will describe the operation as an EmLSCS - Emergency Lower Segment Caesarean Section, or an ElLSCS - Elective Lower Segment Caesarean Section.

Some people would divide the emergency group further, in that these are rarely true emergencies. Most have to be done within an hour or so, but a much smaller number need to be done immediately.

Emergency Caesarean section

If labour is progressing and the baby is becoming distressed but has not passed far enough down the birth canal to be delivered by forceps or Ventouse then the Obstetrician may proceed to a Caesarean section.

There are increasing numbers of Caesarean sections, which is a matter of some concern. It is difficult to find the right solution. We do not want babies to be damaged during labour. This means that once there are signs of a baby being in distress, we will want to speed up the delivery. We don't have a foolproof way of knowing how long it would be safe to let the mother to continue to try and deliver the baby normally, or how long it would take for the baby to be delivered. Because of this we take the 'cautious' approach and do a Caesarean instead.

It would take a brave or perhaps stupid Obstetrician to say 'I think your baby is struggling, but let's leave it to struggle a bit more'.

This means that most babies born even after an emergency Caesarean section come out kicking and screaming.

Caesarean sections with no labour

Because labour prepares the baby for life outside the womb, an elective Caesarean section - that is one without preceding labour means that the baby can be slightly 'caught unawares'. The most significant effect of this is that the baby will not have had any time to prepare for the world outside. Most significantly his lungs will still be filled with 'lung liquid' and this will have to start being cleared from the time of delivery. This usually happens remarkably quickly, but sometimes clearing the fluid from the lungs takes a bit longer and this makes breathing difficult. The baby may need to go to special care for a short while. Once the lungs are cleared, which can take a day or so to complete the baby should be fine and there should be no long-term consequences.

Because elective Caesarean sections often happen before the pregnancy has come to term, they can have some degree of prematurity which may make babies a little more vulnerable. Again, these problems are usually very temporary with no long-term effects, but if we could avoid them that would be even better.

Cerebral palsy

The main reason for all of this is to try and make sure your baby is delivered in good condition. The concern obviously is that if the delivery is difficult this could harm the baby and cause brain damage. The type of damage is usually called cerebral palsy. Unfortunately, we do not know which pregnancies are going to run into trouble. We can say that a particularly pregnancy is low risk or high risk, but this is low risk not no risk. Even the pregnancies considered low risk, need to be monitored because they can occasionally have problems.

Despite our best efforts to improve pregnancy and delivery, children can still develop cerebral palsy. The most likely explanation for this is that whatever causes cerebral palsy can occur during the pregnancy as well as at delivery.

DELIVERY AND AFTER

Now we can concentrate on the star of the show, your baby. As we said by and large your baby won't really mind how he or she is delivered, but will just be pleased to be here. Most of the problems of the newborn period, which seem terrible at the time, are, in reality, little more than blips, which have no long-term significance.

During this time you will be exposed to loads of jargon so I hope that we can prepare you for this a bit, to make you just a teeny bit less neurotic about being a parent than you might otherwise be.

Apgar scores

The Apgar score is a measure of how well the baby is at delivery, or perhaps you might say how well the baby has coped with the effort of being born. The Apgar score measures five different features of wellbeing and is assessed at one minute, five minutes and ten minutes after birth.

One of my favourite questions for students is what does Apgar stand for? Many people think that the five letters represent the five different signs of the score. Actually, I point out, the Apgar score is named after the person who first described it. I then ask who was Apgar and students invariably say that he was a Paediatrician.

Virginia Apgar described the score in 1952, initially as a way of assessing which babies needed resuscitating after birth. It was immensely useful as a way of measuring which drugs given in labour affected the baby and was later on used as a score to predict long-term outcome. We are going to talk about both of these in a minute, but first let's give a few minutes to Professor Apgar. After all, most people who are asked about her think that she must have been a man to have described something famous: amazing how sexist medical education is!

She entered Columbia University in 1929 having already obtained a degree in zoology. She did brilliantly well at medical school and started to train as a surgeon. Although she shone in her surgical training, she was 'advised' against a career as a surgeon because other women had failed to establish themselves, surgery being man's work.

Her boss, seeing that she was full of 'energy, intelligence and ability' encouraged her into the rather neglected field of anaesthetics where she made very significant advances and became the first female professor at Columbia.

She must have been a very formidable lady to achieve what she did despite all the obstacles placed in front of her.

If I can put in a further claim to support my non-sexist credentials, another favourite question regards the Habermann teat, which is a special feeding teat for children with feeding difficulties. Habermann was not a male Paediatrician, but the mother of a baby with poor feeding who would not feed from a normal teat. So, she designed this easy to suck teat, which has revolutionised feeding for thousands of babies.

Alright, let's get back to the Apgar score. As we said, it measures the five characteristics which are in the table, which by chance can be put in order to spell Apgar!

SCORE			
	0	1	2
Activity - muscle tone.	No movement.	Arms and legs flexed.	Moves actively.
Pulse - Heart rate.	Absent.	Less than 100.	More than 100.
Grimace - reflex irritability - response to nasal stimulation.	None.	Grimaces.	Sneezes/ coughs and pulls away.
Appearance - skin colour.	Pale.	Pink body, pale arms and legs.	Pink all over.
Respiration.	Not breathing.	Slow irregular breaths or gasping.	Breathing normally or crying.

So, at one minute, five minutes and ten minutes after birth your baby will be assessed using a chart like this and given a score.

Is it useful?

Yes and no. For many years people have tried to show that the Apgar score predicted how well a baby would do in the future. Those babies with low scores were said to be at a higher risk of long-term problems. Actually most babies with low scores did just fine, it is just that many children with problems had low Apgar scores.

So the Apgar score could let us put babies into different groups. These groups are those with a high Apgar score who have a low risk of long-term problems and those with a low score who have a slightly higher risk of long-term problems. In truth, the Apgar score by itself is never used in this way because, as we said, even if the score is low the outcome is still likely to be OK.

Also, we are a bit more active nowadays. The Apgar score was devised before there was any real treatment for stressed babies, whereas today if we see that a baby looks stressed at delivery we would start treatment immediately. We can also use lots of different tools to judge how stressed they have been and what the chances of long-term damage are. Having said this, most babies are remarkably resilient and although some suffer marked distress, very few of these go on to have long-term problems.

On top of this, ideally the Apgar score should be measured by an independent observer not somebody who is actually involved in looking after the baby. In reality, the midwife or Paediatrician will try to assess the score at the same time as making sure that mother and baby are well, this means that it is often a good guess rather than an accurate measure. And it is much more useful for a baby to be cuddled by his parents as soon as possible than to be dragged away to have an Apgar score taken.

So what is the point?

Being slightly cynical there are two sets of people who remain interested in Apgar scores - midwives and parents. Midwives are obviously anxious that all their babies are born healthy, but beyond this they might have their practice challenged if they deliver a baby who has suffered distress - the argument being that if the baby was in distress the midwife should have called the Obstetrician to deliver the baby instrumentally or by

CaesareanCaesarean section.

So, if a baby is born with low Apgars the midwife can get 'into trouble' and if the baby has high Apgars it proves how good she is.

Similarly, as parents become more and more competitive and place increasing pressure on their children, some of them view the Apgar score as some kind of marker of achievement and future potential. A good Apgar score can be boasted about to show how jolly clever your baby must be.

Because of this, I always try to give as high a score as possible. So if I give a baby Apgar's of 10 and 10 then everybody is happy.

The bottom line, I guess, is that very low Apgar scores identify that a baby has been quite stressed at the time of birth. It isn't anything we can't see for ourselves, but it just gives us a number to use, so that we can feel more scientific.

Neonatal Resuscitation

Most babies come out screaming and do not need any medical attention. They will need to be dried and wrapped to stop them getting too cold and should be quickly given to their parents for a cuddle. Immediately after delivery, a baby's adrenaline levels will be sky high. They will usually be hyper alert and wide eyed. This is a great time for bonding. After half an hour or so, the adrenaline levels fall and the baby will become 'exhausted' and start going to sleep, so it is good to meet your baby as soon as possible.

Occasionally, this will not be possible because your baby may need some medical assistance. All midwives are trained to perform basic neonatal resuscitation and many have much more experience and training. In many hospitals, if your baby needs help then the Paediatrician will be called.

Sometimes a Paediatrician will be called to attend the delivery because the midwives are concerned that your baby is likely to need help. The indications for this will often vary from hospital to hospital but will include such situations as:

- Significant foetal distress
- Baby has passed meconium before delivery
- Instrumental delivery (forceps or Ventouse)
- Emergency Caesarean section

- Problems previously identified with the pregnancy
- Prematurity

On most of these occasions, the baby still comes out kicking and screaming and the Paediatrician is more or less redundant. The midwife may take pity on the Paediatrician and show her the baby first, but will try to get your baby to you as soon as possible.

About 1-2% of babies need a little more help than this. They may need waking up a bit, which can be done by rubbing them down. They may need some oxygen or if they have lots of secretions or meconium about, they may need sucking out. Usually within a few minutes they will be pink and screaming. If this is the case, then there is no evidence that their slow start will have any long term impact whatsoever.

A tiny number of babies, less than 1 in 200, need significant amounts of help. If they do not breathe properly by themselves they may need to have a breathing tube placed in their trachea (windpipe) and then the medical team can take over their breathing for them. If they have a slow heart rate they may need cardiac compressions and if they remain unwell they may need emergency drugs, which would normally be given through a thin tube which is inserted into the umbilical vein - and so is completely painless. Even when babies are this sick, they can still recover well. If you are in this worrying situation, you should feel free to discuss things with the medical team.

Everybody wants to know what the future holds. Unfortunately, we are not great at predicting this. Very occasionally a situation arises where it is clear that a baby will have long term problems, but most of the time we simply cannot tell. One of the challenges of parenthood is trying to enjoy this moment without worrying too much about the next one. Time is the best test for assessing a baby's development and the more milestones they reach at a normal time, the more reassured we are that everything will be alright.

I think we can consider a few different scenarios:

- Nothing has happened that make your baby's chances of being 'normal' any less than any other baby born at term - this applies to most babies that have issues around delivery

- Although it would be better if this had not happened, we have no evidence of any changes that predict long term damage - we have to wait and see and the longer things seem normal the happier we are. This applies to a small number of babies
- There is evidence that what has happened might cause long term problems and so we need to see what these are and try to offer as much treatment or therapy as we can - this happens in less than 0.1% of deliveries

In summary, most babies are born and need no assistance whatsoever. A few do need a little bit of help, but this is normally a minor 'blip' with no long term consequences. Even those that come out quite sick indeed often make an excellent recovery.

The After Birth

First of all, I would like to recap. Information for fathers:

Your partner feels very responsible for your baby - remember that we said that the by-product of conception is guilt. She will have had in her mind an idea of how the whole birthing process was meant to go. It is unlikely that things went to plan. Any slight change or upset will be seen by your partner as a great personal failing which will leave your child forever scarred. She will have forgotten all about the first few chapters of the book which have tried to explain that babies don't much care about the way they are born - they just want to get on and do whatever it is that babies do all day. Remember that your partner will also be feeling tired, exhausted and emotional.

Useful phrases for fathers to cement the parental relationship

- If only you had continued for another few minutes we could have had a normal delivery
- You were making a lot of noise
- Was it really that painful?
- Do you think that's because of the way that she was born?
- In general, support, understanding and thanks are appreciated

---

It's also a rough deal because you as the father might be exhausted, stressed and anxious but nobody will ever ask if you are OK.

Important tips for friends and relatives:

V Few people will actually want to admit that they need help, so ask new parents to call you if they need anything. This way you can more or less guarantee that you will be undisturbed whilst the new parents simply struggle in silence. Don't even think of arriving unannounced with a cooked meal and never ever set to and do the washing or washing up.

Clearly both of you are going to be absorbed, preoccupied and exhausted in the first few weeks. You should accept offers of help as these can make your lives easier. In some communities friends prepare meals for new parents for the first few weeks or so. You might be able to start some sort of reciprocal arrangement with friends/neighbours or antenatal class members. Anybody that visits you and feels that your home is not up to scratch can be given the cleaning stuff or a pot of paint and told to help or get out.

THE 'LET-DOWN' REFLEX

It is easy to fall into the trap of assuming that birth marks the beginning of parenthood or babyhood. You know that it all starts way beforehand. For the baby it usually starts about 9 months beforehand, for the parents it can be even longer.

Most people as they are growing up imagine themselves becoming parents. We develop an idealised picture of our perfect partner, the romance-filled conception followed by a refreshing pregnancy culminating in a normal delivery producing a cherubic child. Sadly, real life is rarely so kind.

When all of these things don't go to plan, it can make us feel disappointed, frustrated, anxious and a whole host of other difficult emotions, which we would prefer not to have to confront. We might call this the 'let down reflex' and it does happen to most of us at some time. If, or more likely when, we feel like this, it can affect the way we think about and relate to, our children, so it is important to try and understand what may be going on.

It is OK to have some mixed feelings about the whole deal of parenthood. I know that you 'would not swap your baby for the world', but you might still miss the weekend lie-ins and lazy days, the socialising and sick-free clothes. The fact that you are now living a completely new life does not mean that you cannot grieve over some of the great bits of your past life which are being drowned in a sea of sterilising fluid and nappies!

Don't feel bad about doing things for yourself. I am neither suggesting nor supporting the idea of abandoning your child, but it is important for your sanity to find some time to escape and also to spend time with your partner and the rest of your family. We all need to find the right balance between 'me-time', 'you-time' and 'us-time'. Think about this as making yourself into a better parent.

If you are feeling frustrated or upset, try to find somebody sympathetic to talk to.

Unhelpful comments to make to exasperated parents:

∇ Well what did you expect?
∇ You wanted a baby in the first place or I don't know why you had that baby.
∇ It was much harder when you were a baby and we didn't have disposable nappies/microwaves/washing machines.
∇ If you had listened to me during the pregnancy you wouldn't be like this now.

Bonding and attachment - It's not always so natural

If you are completely besotted with your baby who is the most amazing wonderful person that you have ever met and you are saying this from a position of strength and you feel privileged just to be on the same planet as this baby and this baby is NOT a comfort for you after, a hard pregnancy, difficult times a bad relationship or a loss; please skip over the next section.

I guess that might leave quite a few people reading on.

Bonding is a very complex phenomenon and can change over time. Like most things, which we will mention, your pre-conceptions, or other people's expectations can make what is actually normal feel like a catastrophe. If the way you are experiencing parenthood is different to what it says in the books - don't worry, it's probably because those books, not you, are wrong.

Most people have different feelings towards their babies at different times, from the positive to the negative. Most of us can acknowledge this and accept that it doesn't make us bad people or failed parents. If you talk openly to other parents you will find that many of them feel exactly the way that you do.

In real life, despite all the turmoil that we go through, we manage to have great relationships with our children. I just want to highlight some issues, which can get in the way a bit. I believe that it is best to acknowledge and address them rather than leave them to fester.

Bonding when the pregnancy is not normal

The heart afraid of breaking...never learns to dance.

Bette Middler "The Rose"

I have spoken to lots of parents, especially mothers who have had scary pregnancies. By this I mean those people who can't quite believe that they are actually going to have a baby. This includes those people who are pregnant after trying for a long time, who have had many miscarriages or have used fertility treatment to get pregnant.

We can add to this list, families who have had some kind of scare during the pregnancy, such as abnormal scans or the onset of premature labour.

The common factor in all of these is the belief that 'I don't want to push my luck. I am not going to have - or don't deserve to have - a normal baby'. Because of this, you believe that the worst is going to happen. Particularly if you have suffered disappointment before, you don't want to raise your hopes too much, to protect yourself a little from the unbearable pain of losing your child.

This is understandable and is a natural defence mechanism. However, it does alter the way that you feel about your unborn baby. Instead of the carefree abandon that many people have during their pregnancy, you are torn between wanting to love your unborn baby and being scared about loving too much. So, your antenatal bonding can be different to what you expected. As we will often mention, as you already feel that everything is your fault, it is very easy to start blaming yourself for the way you feel.

Because antenatal bonding has been altered, you may find that you feel very differently to how you expected to, after your baby is born. You may feel that you are not quite as attached as you think you should be and this makes you feel even worse. You may end up compensating for these feelings by trying to make yourself appear as the most perfect mother ever.

I don't think that I have any answer to this problem. But, I think that recognising that it does exist, even though we wish that it didn't, is a good start. Accepting that it does not make you the devil incarnate or an ungrateful so-and-so, is also important.

Please don't forget that many issues that you may have had beforehand are not necessarily resolved by having a baby. People who have experienced infertility or the loss of babies can still have issues surrounding these tragedies. They do not go away just because you have a baby, but need confronting and resolving as separate issues.

Bonding and the premature baby

A lot has been written about whether having a premature baby affects bonding. Some of the ideas are the same as those we have just mentioned, as many babies born prematurely have had less than straightforward pregnancies. There is then the added guilt of feeling that you have failed your baby by not being able to carry them to term and the anxiety, often misplaced that your baby may not survive or have long-term problems. All of these are normal feelings, which need to be acknowledged.

I was referred an eight year old girl who had some very minor problems, but was actually a wonderful child. Her mother was very concerned about her health and development, which were effectively normal. As she was born at 28 weeks gestation this was a brilliant outcome. After a few minutes it became clear that the essence of the problem was that her mother was still overcome by guilt at going into premature labour. Trying to compensate for having failed her daughter so terribly had distorted their relationship. If the daughter had any problems then they must be the result of the prematurity, which was the mother's fault. So she was, at the same time both desperately looking for problems and wishing that they did not exist.

Not surprisingly, her husband was happy that the problem was his wife's. He was less impressed when I pointed out that the fact that his wife had carried this, without his support or interest for the last nine years, meant that they must have some issues too.

Added to all of this, it can be hard to feel that the baby on a neonatal unit is actually yours. It seems that you are just a visitor who is sometimes invited in to do a few tasks. Tasks like feeding and changing your baby, which should belong to you, you now can only do with permission. Most neonatal units do not have much privacy; this often makes people too embarrassed to do simple grown-up things like singing to or dancing with babies. There is also, as one mother said, 'a limit to what you can say to a premature baby in an incubator when you are surrounded by nurses!'

Bonding - Danger signs

There is clearly a whole range of normal bonding from the obsessive to the near indifferent. This will fluctuate somewhat throughout your life.

Many mothers have inexplicable mood changes after pregnancy these range from the so called 'baby blues' through postnatal depression to the severe 'puerperal psychosis'. One of the results of these conditions could be bonding failure, or more alarmingly having unpleasant thoughts about your baby or a feeling of wanting to harm your baby. If you are feeling like this it is vital that you don't ignore it. For everybody's sake please speak to your midwife or doctor as soon as possible.

THE MAIN ATTRACTION

That's enough talking about you; let's get back to serious things like your baby. We will look at what is important in the first hours, days and weeks of your baby's life. We will also look briefly at what happens if there are any slip ups, although there is more information on these in the section on the neonatal unit.

Being born is hard work, especially if you have had a normal delivery. In fact the whole event is a lot more stressful for your baby than it is for you. You have to cope with being a new parent but your baby has to cope with much more. He has to get used to a whole new way of life, from being swaddled in the warm dark comfort of the womb he has to learn to live in the cold, light world outside. No more is everything done for him through the placenta. He has to start breathing and keep on doing it - using his lungs to breathe. He needs to feed for himself and keep himself warm; he needs to have a generally high level of alertness.

The essentials for a baby are:

- Breathing
- Eating
- Keeping his temperature up

An essential component to respiration is the baby changing from a circulation in the womb where oxygen is delivered by the placenta directly to the body, to one where it is delivered by breathing air into the lungs. At birth babies' oxygen levels will usually be a little low and they may look blue. They should start breathing immediately and turn pink within a few minutes.

Sometimes as a result of a very stressful delivery, they can be born 'out of breath' and will breathe very quickly to blow off the acid that has built up during delivery.

Very occasionally a baby might need help breathing. Reasons for this include:

- Being born prematurely
- Inhaling meconium
- Being extremely stressed
- Born too quickly - with not enough time to empty their lungs before being born
- Having a Chest infection or heart problem

Although this list looks quite scary, these are rare events and invariably babies respond well to treatment with no long term consequences.

Feeding

Most babies do not feed loads in the first few days of life and they have enough reserves to tide them over until feeding kicks off on about the third day of life. If you are breast feeding, this is about the same time that your milk will start to come through. The most important part of feeding is to make sure that the blood sugar levels do not fall. A low blood sugar level can be dangerous for a baby, because if the brain is not supplied with enough sugar it can sustain damage. For most babies this is never a problem, but there are some babies who might need some extra help.

Babies that have had a degree of placental insufficiency and are born relatively small will not have had enough energy supply in the womb to lay down energy stores. After delivery they will need to ensure a good energy supply.

Another group are babies whose mothers have diabetes. In this situation, because the mother's blood sugars are high, the baby is exposed to excess sugar in the womb. As a response to this he will produce an increased amount of insulin. Insulin is a hormone which, among other things works to reduce the amount of sugar in the blood. After birth, when the supply of extra sugar falls - because the baby is no longer connected to the placenta, the baby will still continue to produce the insulin for a while. This can make his blood sugar drop quite seriously.

These babies may have their blood sugars checked soon after birth and a more intense feeding plan put in place. For most babies this will just entail asking you to feed them a little more, particularly than might otherwise be the case. If despite this the sugar levels keep falling, they may need to be fed through a tube or drip until their sugar levels are maintained at a safe level. For most babies this is only an issue for a few days.

The medical term for blood sugar is blood glucose and we call a low blood sugar hypoglycaemia. It is easy to measure the blood glucose using a drop of blood on a special test strip. Lots of doctors and nurses will refer to the blood sugar as the 'BM'. BM does not mean anything; it is just the initials of Boehringer Mannheim, the trade name of one of the popular testing strips!

Temperature control

It is normal for babies' temperatures to drop a little immediately after birth. Cooling the body after stress can reduce or prevent damage to the body's organs. Increasingly this is being used in all fields of medicine to reduce brain and heart damage. Because delivery can be stressful, nature allows a baby to cool a little bit to help protect their vital organs.

However, getting too cold (hypothermia) or being cold for too long is not good for a normal baby. This is for a few reasons. Essentially our bodies do not work as well at low temperatures and if a baby gets cold he will use up energy trying to keep up his temperature and this may leave very little energy to do other things.

Because staying warm is so important, your baby will be dried straight after delivery and wrapped up in a few blankets. If he is unable to keep warm by himself, then he may need extra wrapping or being placed under a heater. Sometimes getting cold can be a sign of infection, so if your baby is persistently cold it would be normal for them be examined by a midwife or Paediatrician.

Vitamin K

If you think your baby is perfect on the outside, you would be even more impressed if you think about how he actually 'works'. The human body is an unbelievable feat of engineering. For example, blood has to be able to flow freely through the blood vessels, but if these vessels are damaged it has to be able to limit how much blood is lost. If the blood is too 'thick' it will start sludging and blocking up the blood vessels, which will mean that the blood supply to the organs is impaired. If it does not clot easily enough, then there will be easy and often prolonged bleeding.

In simple cases, this could just mean that if you cut yourself it will take a longer time for it to stop bleeding. More worryingly, in some cases a little knock or change could cause catastrophic internal bleeding.

Vitamin K is very important in the production of a number of substances that help the blood clot (Clotting Factors). A tiny number of babies do not seem to have enough of these clotting factors and so are susceptible to having significant bleeding which can be life changing or life threatening. This is called Haemorrhagic Disease of the Newborn. Because it is impossible to know which babies are susceptible to this, it seems sensible to give every baby vitamin K when they are born. No baby who has received an adequate dose of vitamin K has had any serious bleeding.

The most efficient way to give vitamin K is as a single injection. It can also be given orally - normally as three doses. Unfortunately, about 20 years ago, there was a scare about the safety of vitamin K. As normally happens in these situations parents refused vitamin K for their children, more children had serious bleeds and a few years later the scare was shown to be without foundation.

I do not know any Paediatricians who would not give their children Vitamin K as an injection.

WHAT HAPPENS NEXT?

Okay. So you now have gone through probably the most amazing experience of your life. You have created this amazing new person. You are exhilarated and exhausted. On one hand you probably feel that you no longer own your own body considering how much it has been prodded and inspected by the world and his wife, whilst on the other hand you wish that somebody else did own your body, seeing how sore it is.

What you need now as a mother is cosseting, caring, appreciation, recognition and celebration. The problem is where are you going to get it from? I am going to be brutally honest. Unfortunately, midwifery services are so stretched that it is hard to guarantee that you will receive it from an NHS postnatal ward. If possible you should have a back-up plan. Do not be afraid to ask for help. Visitors who help should be made welcome, especially those that you can ask to leave.

There will be times - from now on and forever when you will want to be alone with your baby and do things by yourself and there may be times when you are so desperate that you would entrust your child to some ravenous flesh eating monster. Everybody will want to cuddle your baby and this again can make you feel different things - such as pride, pleasure and jealousy - perhaps all at the same time.

You may also feel a loss of control. Well meaning relatives may mistake you for your baby and infantilise you whilst taking control of the situation. You may welcome and resent this at the same time. Take solace. If things go to plan then in one generation's time you will be able to inflict the same burden on your own children.

At this stage it is important to think about the poor father, somewhat a peripheral player. Men, in general, so I am frequently reminded, suffer from being quite useless. They have very rudimentary communication skills and if they do identify an emotion, rarely possess any effective way of articulating this. Unfortunately, this means that they are often overlooked. They have had to play second fiddle to their partner who has done all the 'hard work' and are now playing third fiddle because mother and baby come first. Please remember that however primitive we may be, men have needs too.

EXAMINATION OF THE NEWBORN - THE BABY CHECK

Assuming everything goes to plan, the next major medical hurdle for your baby will be the newborn examination. At birth, the first checks will take place, making sure that your baby has the requisite numbers of things in more or less the right place. Later on, sometime between about six hours and a week, your baby will have a further medical check.

This is in many ways a 'quality control' check, trying to identify if there are any problems that are likely to need addressing. Although I will refer to a doctor examining your child, the check could be performed by your GP, a trained midwife or a Paediatrician. The check is often done in hospital before you go home, but it is not a discharge examination. And if your baby is well, they can be discharged home and have a newborn examination in the next few days. We will discuss what is involved in the check and what it can and can't do. There are a number of things that need to be looked for during the examination - a checklist. Because the examination will depend on how co-operative your baby is the examination may have to be tailored to get everything in at your baby's convenience.

Antenatal History:

The doctor examining your baby should find out what has been happening to your baby over the last 9 months. This will include finding out about your scans, blood tests and any medications that you have been on. They should also discuss if you or any family members have any medical problems, which could be relevant to your baby.

General Wellbeing:

If you are happy with your baby, your baby has fed, passed urine and meconium, settled and woken up, then these are all wonderful signs and indicate that most systems are working well.

General Appearance:

How does your baby look? Obviously we all look different, but there are some conditions where babies have a very typical appearance. Having said that, sometimes changes can be subtle and hard to pick up.

Another thing to look for is your baby's colour. Are they nice and pink or do they look jaundiced. Babies with heart or breathing problems may look blue.

Do they have the right things in the right places; fingers, toes, eyes etc.

Skin:

Making sure that there are no rashes or signs of infection.

Skull and Nervous System:

The doctor will feel your baby's skull and check that the fontanelles - soft spots - are normal. A baby will usually have two, one at the top of the head - the anterior fontanelle, which is usually diamond shaped and a smaller triangular one - the posterior fontanelle towards the back of the skull.

The size of the fontanelles is rarely of importance. The anterior fontanelle can vary from 0.5 to about 5 cm (1/4 inch to 2 inches) across. There are many myths about fontanelles. They are not more sensitive than any other part of the skin and I don't think anybody has ever accidentally pushed a finger through one - they are not especially fragile. Although most babies have two, in some conditions babies can have extra fontanelles.

As well as feeling the fontanelles, the doctor will feel the sutures on the skull. A baby's skull is made of a number of different bones, which are not joined together; the sutures are where the skull bones meet each other. The sutures and fontanelles are important as the skull needs to be able to cope with the rapid brain growth which takes place in the first few years of life. The sutures and fontanelles give the brain some leeway to expand as required. As children get older, these bones join together (fuse) to form, in effect, a single bone. In some conditions the bones are joined prematurely.

The doctor should also record your baby's head circumference - the size of the head and look to see if there is any bruising after delivery. It is not unusual for a baby's head to be a bit squashed after delivery, but this normally corrects itself over the course of a few days or weeks.

There is a limited examination of the nervous system, which checks that everything is in order. The first part of this is observing how your baby reacts. Does he seem to respond, does he move his arms and legs normally, does he wake to feed and feed alright.

The examination will include lifting your baby up to check his tone. Your baby should be a bit, but not too floppy as the doctor holds him as if he is lying on his tummy. The doctor will also check that your baby can suck properly and look for some basic reflexes. These include the Moro reflex. Sometimes this can look a little careless - but it is intended to be part of the check. If your baby falls back a little bit, he should stretch out his arms and then bring them together. Other reflexes, which are usually more pleasing to watch, are walking and stepping reflexes, where your baby will make walking movements or look like he is trying to climb a step and the Grasp reflex when your baby will try to grip on to a finger that is placed in his palm or on the sole of his feet.

Your baby's eyes should also be checked. This is very limited, but involves shining a light into his eyes. The doctor should be able to see the red-reflex. This is like getting a red-eye on a flash photograph. In some eye problems the red reflex is absent.

Gastrointestinal System:

A lot of this can be checked from the history of feeding and passing meconium. The doctor will want to check your baby's palate - the roof of the mouth. If there is any gap in the palate, this will require treatment and may cause short term feeding problems. The doctor will also feel your baby's tummy and check his bottom, to make sure that the anus is in the right position.

Heart/Cardiovascular System:

As we have mentioned above, after birth your baby has to change from living in the womb to living in the outside world. The plumbing of the heart is different for both situations and fully switching over can take a few days. The main change is that blood having bypassed the lungs now has to go through the lungs. In order to achieve this, a connection between the left and right side of the heart has to close, as does a blood vessel that connects the main blood vessel of the body, the aorta to the main blood vessel to the lungs - the pulmonary artery. At the same time the blood pressure in the lungs drops from being higher than the blood pressure in the rest of the body, to being much lower.

A heart murmur occurs when there is abnormal flow of blood. Because of the changes mentioned above, many babies will have murmurs in the first few hours of life as the pre-birth channels close. Also, some heart murmurs will only become noticeable after a few days. This is because even if there is an abnormal connection, if the pressures on both sides of it are the same, there will not be any flow through it. Once the pressure on one side falls, then blood will flow through the connection and a murmur will be able to be heard with a stethoscope. This is one of the reasons why your baby will be rechecked when he is around six weeks old. Heart murmurs are quite common - and occur in over 2% of babies. Most of the time they are benign and do not represent any serious heart problem. Often as the heart grows small defects improve. If your baby does have a heart murmur, then he is likely to be examined by a number of different doctors. He may well have an ECG - looking at the electrical activity of the heart, which is of limited value and an X-Ray, which is of even more limited value.

Usually, he will be re-examined after a few days or weeks, in most cases the murmur will have disappeared. If it persists it is likely that he will have an echocardiogram, which is an ultrasound scan of the heart. This is a test that requires a lot of skill, so your baby may need to be referred to another hospital.

Most babies with significant heart problems will be identified during antenatal ultrasound scanning, but a few will slip through the net. If your baby has any of the following symptoms then you should seek urgent advice.

- Looks blue
- Sweating
- Breathing fast
- Poor feeding - especially if he sweats or pants during feeds

Respiratory System:

There is a limit to how much this can be examined. If your baby is pink and breathing easily then this essentially rules out any significant problems.

Abdomen:

The doctor will look at your baby's tummy and check to make sure that the internal organs are not enlarged. Because most babies have had ultrasound scans during the pregnancy, it is rare to find anything unexpected during the postnatal exam.

Hernias:

A hernia is a protrusion or 'sticking out'. It happens if the internal organs, usually the intestines or the fat covering them, pops out through a gap in the abdominal muscles. The two types of hernia seen most often in children are those around the belly button - umbilical hernias, or in the groin - inguinal hernias.

Umbilical hernias are not uncommon - particularly in black babies. They can vary in size from the size of a fingertip to the size of the child's fist. They are caused by a temporary weakness in the muscles of the abdomen which allows a bit of bowel or some fat to stick out. They will get bigger and harder as the baby cries. They are completely harmless and will not be a cause of pain. They tend to get smaller and usually disappear after a few years. Very occasionally they may need surgery. The old wives' suggestion of binding an old penny over them has no merit whatsoever.

Occasionally an umbilical hernia can be linked to other problems - such as an underactive thyroid gland. This would in any case be tested for with the blood test taken at a few days of age. Other conditions should be obvious and very few babies with umbilical hernias need any investigations or treatment.

Inguinal hernias are much rarer and can be difficult to detect. They are much more common in boys than in girls. In boys they can appear as a lump in the groin or - a swelling in the scrotal sac. This is because in the foetus, the testes start off in the abdomen and drop down into the scrotum. The path that they create can sometimes be open enough for a hernia to slip through. Some boys are born with hydroceles (water on the testicles) which usually disappear over the first few weeks or months of life. Distinguishing a hernia from a hydrocele can be quite hard.

If a hernia is detected, the boy will need an operation to replace it and to close the gap which it fell through so that it can't drop out again. This is done as a routine procedure. However, occasionally a hernia can get stuck or incarcerated. If this happens the bowel in the hernia can lose its blood supply and this can be very painful and dangerous. Any child with a hernia who seems unsettled or unwell - particularly if they are vomiting should be checked immediately and may need urgent surgery.

Genitalia:

If you have a boy, it is important to check that the penis looks normal. Occasionally the urethra - the opening does not open at the right place. This may need an operation later on. In that case, there is no need for alarm, but the foreskin may need to be used in the operation and if you were going to circumcise your son, then you should delay it until he has been seen by the surgeon.

The other important thing in boys is to see the urinary stream. Most boys should be able to 'hit you in the eye'. If they have more of an old man's dribble then they may have a urinary blockage, which will need speedy treatment.

In most boys both testicles can be felt in the scrotum. If they are not there yet, they are likely to come down over the next few months. Rarely, if they do not come down by themselves they will need an operation to help bring them down. If the testicles cannot be felt, this will need to be monitored.

As mentioned above, some boys have some fluid on the testicles - a hydrocele. This in itself is of little significance and will normally disappear. For those that seem to persist for a long time, a small operation may be required.

Girls are always much simpler and it is extremely rare to find any problems. Occasionally they may have small skin tags on the vagina. These do not normally need any treatment. It is not unusual for girls to have a small amount of vaginal discharge, which can be bloodstained. This happens because having been exposed to their mothers hormones in the womb, these are now removed and the baby can have some 'breakthrough bleeding'. This can last for a few days and is not a cause for concern.

Similarly, they may produce small quantities of 'milk' from their breasts.

Hips:

The hip is described as a 'ball and socket type joint' as the thigh bone (femur) fits into the pelvic bone (acetabulum) like a ball into a socket. Rarely this joint does not form properly, making the hip either dislocated - where the thigh bone is outside the pelvis, or easily dislocatable. Early treatment of this is usually straightforward and highly successful. However, if diagnosis is delayed, the treatment will be more invasive and less likely to be fully successful. To check the stability of your baby's hips, the doctor will perform a few manoeuvres on them. These may be a little uncomfortable for your baby.

Most babies will not have any problems during this check. Because doctors will want to be certain, if there is any doubt it is quite common for them to ask for a second opinion. Most of the time, the more experienced doctor will decide that your baby is fine.

COMMON PROBLEMS ON THE POSTNATAL WARD

Even healthy babies can have a few hiccups in the first few days of life. Like most things that we discuss these are more likely to upset you than they are to upset your baby.

Birth Trauma

This is common - especially if your baby has had a difficult delivery. Some 'moulding' of the skull is common even after a normal delivery, when the head can look both squashed and swollen. This is likely to settle down over the first few days or so. If your baby has been born by forceps or Ventouse, they may have not only moulding from the period of labour before delivery, but also some trauma from the delivery.

Although the Obstetrician will try to be as gentle as possible whilst delivering your baby by forceps or Ventouse, they often need to use quite a bit of force. This can cause some local swelling or scarring, but however horrible these may look at the beginning, they will clear up completely. Sometimes if a delivery has been very difficult, your baby may even have a small skull fracture. This definitely sounds more horrible than it is, as it is likely to not bother your baby at all and again will heal completely.

Very big babies may break their collar bones (clavicle) during delivery. Often this can go unnoticed, although a baby with a broken collar bone may not like having the arm on the affected side moved and may be a little grizzly. Similarly, babies can get nerve injuries. The most common of these is a so-called 'Erbs Palsy'. This results in the baby holding the arm in a slightly strange position (the waiters tip position). Whilst this injury usually improves over time, physiotherapy input can be useful.

A further fairly common presentation is a baby with a 'stiff neck', or torticollis. Here the neck is tilted to one side or the baby seems reluctant to look to the other side. This can be caused by a swelling in the main muscle that goes from the head to the front of the body. It is thought that damage to the muscle, such as a small tear can cause a bleed into the muscle. This causes a swelling, which makes muscle movement more difficult. Just to scare you we call this a 'sterno-cleido-mastoid tumour'. The sterno-cleido-mastoid is the name of the muscle and tumour just means swelling. This condition has nothing whatsoever to do with cancer. It resolves over time. Basic advice is to try and position and interact with your baby so that they will have to use their weaker side. Sometimes physiotherapy is needed as well.

Erythema Toxicum Neonatorum - blotchy baby

About a third of babies will develop a rash over the first few days of life. This can look very angry. Usually there are little, pinhead sized, white spots - like tiny spots of acne with a surrounding area of redness, which can spread out quite a long way. They can often more or less cover the whole of the body. Although it can look very frightening it is completely harmless and will settle in a few days. No treatment is required.

It is thought the rash is caused by a reaction in the skin to normal bacteria. The womb is a wonderfully clean place and should be completely sterile. After birth our skin is covered or colonised by bacteria, which are usually harmless. When the bacteria first come into contact with the skin, there may be a reaction, which gives the rash.

The rash can look very dramatic and sometimes even midwives may be taken aback by this. This leads to the classic ironic situation where parents and midwives are concerned. They will call the doctor saying 'can you come and see this baby who has an angry looking red rash?' The doctor will arrive, take a look and intone,'Ah yes, that's Erythema Toxicum Neonatorum'. It sounds very impressive until you realise that Erythema Toxicum Neonatorum is just Latin for an 'Angry red rash that babies get'.

Occasionally babies can get a more serious skin infection, especially around the umbilicus. In this case, they will usually need antibiotics.

Birth Marks

Birth marks are common - and are not always present at birth. We will briefly discuss a few of the most common ones. More information is available from the Birthmark Support Group Tel: 0845 045 4700 www.birthmarksupportgroup.org.uk

Stork Mark: These occur in about 50% of babies, often on the forehead or neck. They look a group of little red spots. They are completely harmless and usually fade over the first few years of life.

Mongolian blue spots: are extremely common, especially in Black and Asian babies. They are flat, bluish grey marks. They can appear in any area and babies can have quite a few of them. They often appear on or near the buttocks and usually disappear after a few years. Although they are entirely benign, they can sometimes be mistaken as bruises. Unfortunately, some babies are even referred to social services, because somebody mistakes a Mongolian blue spot for a bruise. This just creates unnecessary worry and anxiety. So, if your baby has a Mongolian blue spot ask somebody to document it in their records to help avoid any confusion later on.

Milia (milk spots): These are tiny white spots, which often appear on the face, they can look a bit like heat rash. Again they are of no concern and will disappear over time.

Strawberry marks: These are often not present at birth but develop over the first few weeks. They can appear anywhere and can be of any size. They look raised and red - probably more raspberry than strawberry colour. They increase in size over a few months and then fade over the next few years. They often leave a bit of a mark behind. Usually they are harmless. They can pose problems if they are in a difficult area or if they are very large or there are loads of them. Occasionally these birthmarks can grow in difficult areas, for example close to the eye. They could then obstruct a baby's vision and would need treatment. Other problems arise if the strawberry mark is massive, not only can it look unsightly, but sometimes a lot of blood and platelets can get 'trapped' in the birthmarks which affects overall blood clotting. This can also happen if there are many smaller ones.

In all of the above situations, when there is a medical need for treatment, this can be performed at specialist centres. Normally it would entail laser therapy to the birthmark or injecting drugs that help make it smaller. Strawberry marks that are harmless are normally left alone, as treatment is likely to do more harm than good. As treatments develop over the years, it might well be that this balance will change.

The natural history of strawberry marks is that they increase in size for 6-12 months before getting smaller. They are painless, but can sometimes bleed and scab over a bit. This is not dangerous and just needs simple treatment.

Port wine stain: This is a much rarer birthmark and normally occurs on the forehead. It is usually flat and dark red - hence it's name. There can be a link with port wine stains and other abnormalities, so a baby with one of these will normally have a number of other investigations.

Seborrhea/ Cradle cap: This can look quite unpleasant. It is caused by blocked glands and can make the skin look spotted and greasy. It is completely harmless and usually improves with time.

In cradle cap the scalp can look sore and it seems as if the skin is flaking off. Again, this is unlikely to bother your baby although it can look nasty. The simplest remedy is to wash your babies head every day or so using olive oil, or something similar.

Jaundice

Jaundice (yellowing of the skin) is inevitable in every baby. It is caused by a high level of bilirubin, which is formed by the breakdown of haemoglobin in red blood cells. The bilirubin is processed (conjugated) in the liver to a form which allows it to be passed out of the body via the bowels. There must be some benefit to babies in having a high bilirubin soon after birth, but there is little agreement as to what this is. One suggestion is that bilirubin is an anti-oxidant and is useful for helping to mop up the oxidants that are formed by the stress of delivery.

Essentially, as mentioned above babies have proportionally more red blood cells than adults - their blood is 'thicker'. Blood cells, like many cells in the body, last for a certain period of time and then 'die' and are replaced by new ones. Babies' blood cells have a shorter turnover time, so don't last as long. This means that there is increased red cell destruction and production of bilirubin. Added to this, a baby's liver may not be able to process the bilirubin as well as an adult could, which would make the levels remain high. Breast-feeding seems to make jaundice deeper and last longer. Although this has been known about for centuries, nobody fully understands why this should be. It is probably due to the fact that some of the hormones or chemicals in breast milk interfere with the passing out of bilirubin from the body. Despite this, there is rarely, if ever, a reason why breast-feeding should stop because of jaundice.

Types and causes of Jaundice:

Basically, there are two 'types' of jaundice. Before the bilirubin is processed by the liver it is said to be 'unconjugated', this type of bilirubin can cross into the brain and if the levels are extremely high can cause brain damage. Once the bilirubin has been processed by the liver it becomes 'conjugated' in this form it can not enter into the brain, but a high level of conjugated bilirubin can be a sign of significant liver disease.

Normally, jaundice becomes visible after a few days, reaches a peak and then fades slowly over a few days to weeks. It is more likely than not that a baby will have some level of jaundice. But there are some instances when we take jaundice seriously and this depends on: the time it starts, the level of jaundice and the type. If a baby seems to be significantly jaundiced then we need to treat the jaundice to stop the level getting too high and try to find out what the cause is.

If the level of bilirubin rises, it begins to become visible in the body. At slightly raised levels, it is first evident by the whites of the eyes becoming a bit yellow. At higher levels, the skin begins to look yellow. There is probably some truth in the observation that as jaundice becomes more severe, more parts of the body are affected. Initially just the head, at higher levels the head and body and at even higher levels the whole body to the tips of the fingers and toes. Unfortunately, this is not entirely reliable and the only real way to asses jaundice is by measuring the level. It is certainly very difficult to assess babies who are not white skinned and normally any black or Asian baby who is visibly jaundiced should have this checked.

Nowadays, there are some machines that can measure jaundice levels through the skin. These are not entirely accurate and not used everywhere. In many places, the only way to measure jaundice is by a blood test.

The level of jaundice that merits concern depends on a number of factors, especially the gestation of the baby and how old they are. In the UK, there are now unified charts, which help direct appropriate management of jaundice. By way of confusion there are different ways of measuring the levels. The UK uses a different system to America. (For the record the American 1mg/dL is the same as the English 17 micromols/l, so a level of 20 in America is the same as 340 in England).

If a baby has a significant level of jaundice, then we need to identify a cause and treat the jaundice. Identifying the cause may include blood tests and occasionally other investigations. Treatment options include, ensuring that the baby is well hydrated, the use of special light - either as an overhead light or a blanket, the use of some drugs and blood transfusions.

The principle of phototherapy (light treatment) is that the light rays pass through the skin and turn the fat soluble bilirubin into a water soluble bilirubin. Whilst it is fat soluble it can enter the brain, but can't be passed in urine, or very much in stool. If it is made water soluble it is less toxic, can't pass into the brain and can be passed in stool more easily. Phototherapy has been extremely widely used for many decades and appears to be incredibly safe. As a precaution, a baby will have his eyes shielded by an eye mask. It is helpful to keep the baby as exposed as possible, because the more skin that absorbs the light, the quicker the levels will go down. Obviously, if a baby does need phototherapy, keeping him exposed to the light is important but this should not prevent feeding or cuddling.

Unfortunately, you can't use any type of light; the light is UV-B light. It is present in sunlight, but it is not advisable to expose a baby to excessive sunlight, because of the risk of sunburn. The light can be provided by overhead lights, which are very effective, but often make it feel as if your baby is inaccessible. The light can make your baby look a strange blue whilst under it.

Increasingly light producing sheets (bili-blankets) are used and these seem less intrusive. Once treatment is started, the bilirubin levels will need to be checked to make sure that the treatment is effective. Once the levels have fallen the lights can be stopped. It would be normal to check this at least one more time, to make sure that the bilirubin level has not bounced back up again.

There are other potential treatments for jaundice. However, because they are 'low-tech' and freely available, there is little opportunity for any company to make any money out of them. Because most medical research is profit motivated, there are no funds available to give these treatments proper trials. The NICE guidelines on neonatal jaundice say that alternative treatments for jaundice cannot be recommended because there is not enough evidence to show that they work and don't have side effects. At present it seems as if phototherapy is the only option.

Jaundice noted on the first day of life (rhesus disease):

It usually takes a day or so for jaundice to become noticeable. Jaundice, which is evident before this time could be linked to a medical problem. It is likely that if your baby is jaundiced during this time, he will need some investigations. The most important cause of early jaundice is a rapid breakdown of red blood cells (haemolysis). This can happen for a number of reasons, but in the first day of life, it is important to consider a condition called 'haemolytic disease of the newborn' or 'rhesus disease'.

Your type of blood group is genetically determined. That is, it depends on your parents' blood groups. If blood from a different blood group enters your blood stream, you will make antibodies against it, which will destroy the 'foreign' blood. Although a mother and baby do not share the same blood, sometimes a baby's blood can leak from the placenta into the mother's blood stream. This could happen during a medical procedure on the baby, or if whilst pregnant you get hit or knocked on the abdomen.

When a baby and mother are of different blood groups, if the baby's blood enters the mother's blood stream it will cause her to make antibodies against it. There are numerous possibilities for this mismatch to happen. Blood is grouped into three main groups A, B and O. the next main division is into rhesus groups, positive or negative. The most common mismatch is when a rhesus negative mother has a rhesus positive baby. If the mother is exposed to the baby's blood she can start to make antibodies to it. Once these are created they essentially last for ever and so can cause problems in not only the current pregnancy but also future pregnancies.

Antibodies are useful in fighting infections and they cross over the placenta from the mother to the baby. This is usually helpful to the baby, because it means that after birth the baby has some protection against a number of infections. However, if the mother is making antibodies to her baby's blood, these will cross over into the baby and cause destruction of some of the baby's blood cells (haemolysis).

This is why mothers have their blood groups tested in early pregnancy; because if they are rhesus negative they are treated as if there babies are rhesus positive. At any time when there is a possibility of babies blood entering into the mothers blood stream, she should receive an injection (of Rhesus anti-D) antibodies that will mop up the babies blood cells in the mothers system before they trigger her to make her own response.

Sometimes a rhesus negative mother will be sensitised without knowing it, or there may be other blood incompatibilities which we are not able to test for. If this happens, the rapid destruction of red cells causes both an increase in the amount of bilirubin produced and can also cause anaemia. Severe cases will normally be picked up before delivery, because significant anaemia in a foetus cause specific ultrasound changes and occasionally a baby might need blood transfusions whilst still in the womb.

Less severe cases can be detected after birth. It is important to start early treatment. Treatment involves not only making sure that the jaundice level does not become dangerously high, but may also involve treating the cause. As the cause is the presence of antibodies in the baby's blood, the best way to deal with this is by doing a blood exchange and replacing the baby's blood through a transfusion.

There are other causes of haemolysis (rapid breakdown of red blood cells). These are usually caused by genetic problems which cause the cells to have abnormal shapes, or where some important enzymes in the cells are missing. The most important of these is known as G6PD (Glucose-6-Phosphate Dehydrogenase). G6PD is an important anti-oxidant in red blood cells. When there is not enough G6PD this means that the red blood cells are particularly fragile. The appropriate trigger can cause rapid haemolysis which can be dangerous not only because of the jaundice caused but also because of the rapid loss of blood cells.

G6PD deficiency is rare in the white British population, but is quite common in people of Mediterranean, Asian or African descent. In the newborn period it can present with severe jaundice in the first week or so of life. Although there is no treatment for G6PD deficiency it is important to diagnose, so that you can try to prevent 'haemolytic crises' by avoiding those things known to trigger them.

Other conditions, such as thalassaemia and sickle cell disease will not cause problems until a few months of age.

Jaundice noted between 1 day and two weeks:

As mentioned above, almost all babies will have some degree of jaundice in the first few weeks of life. As long as your baby is feeding well and behaving normally and the jaundice does not seem too severe, no action will normally be required. If your baby is not feeding well or seems unwell or quite deeply jaundiced, then it is likely that he will need to undergo some tests.

Obviously, the first test would be to check the level of the jaundice. If this seems high, your baby will need this to be treated regardless of what the cause is.

Other tests will check to make sure that your baby does not have an infection, that his blood count is alright and that his liver is working alright. Sometimes, if there is any doubt, your baby may be given antibiotics as a precaution. We will discuss this in more detail when we talk about infections.

Persistent jaundice:

Although jaundice can persist for many months, especially in breast fed babies, in most babies it will have virtually disappeared by a few weeks of age. Most importantly, there is an extremely rare liver disease called biliary atresia, which occurs in babies. It presents with jaundice and gets progressively more serious over a short period of time. If it is detected and treated early, within six weeks, there is an excellent outcome, but if treatment is delayed, there is a risk of long term irreversible and progressive liver damage.

So, although it is a condition that only affects about one baby in 10,000. It is serious enough for us to want to catch every case early. Because of this we like to review every baby who is still jaundiced at around two weeks of age. The jaundice in biliary atresia is a different type of jaundice to the usual one, in that the bilirubin has been processed by the liver. This means that babies with biliary atresia have a greenish look to them.

Another result of this condition is that the urine looks dark and the stool is light (de-pigmented). A baby's urine should be clear and colourless and their stools should be a green or bright yellow colour. There are excellent colour charts available from www.childliverdisease.org look for the 'stool colour bookmark'.

If your baby is jaundiced at two weeks of age, they should be assessed. This will include checking feeding and growth and a physical examination. In the UK most children will have a blood test, to measure the total bilirubin level and to see whether the bilirubin is the type that is linked to liver problems. In other countries of the world, they may use the stool charts. In either case, the overwhelming majority of children that are tested merely have persisting 'normal' jaundice.

Infection - Sepsis

The most common reason for a newborn baby to receive medical attention is the concern that they may have an infection. Up to 10% of normal healthy babies will be examined for a possible infection. Of these only a tiny proportion will actually have an infection, but most if not all will receive treatment.

Paediatricians are paranoid about infections in babies. This is because babies, who have only subtle signs to suggest that they may be unwell, may actually be brewing something very nasty. They can then deteriorate rapidly, getting extremely sick. Because of this we don't like taking any chances and if there is any suspicion of an infection in babies less than a few weeks old, most Paediatricians in the world would advise that treatment should be started. This means that we treat many more babies than is necessary, but we do not have any guaranteed way of establishing which babies we need to treat and which we could safely leave.

Most of medical practice is based on experience and to challenge that experience we conduct clinical trials to see if a new treatment is better than an existing one, or whether any treatment is needed at all. In order to carry out these trials, we need one group of patients who will not receive the current treatment. If we were to perform trials to see if there were babies that definitely did not need antibiotics when there was a suspicion of an infection, this would mean that a group of these babies would not get treatment. Most Paediatricians would feel uncomfortable with this. So we just treat them.

All of this means that we have a very low threshold for considering and treating possible infections in babies. It means that we probably treat about 100 babies just in case one of them has a serious infection. At present it looks like this is going to continue, because that 1% chance is not worth taking.

The womb is a sterile environment, as long as the membranes remain intact. If the membranes rupture - the waters break - then the womb becomes vulnerable. Indeed, infection is a cause for the membranes rupturing in the first place. A number of infections can get into the womb, normally ascending via the birth canal. Once inside the womb germs can multiply and cause infection. The longer the waters have been broken for, the greater is the likelihood that bacteria will enter and grow inside it. In general the risk is very small in the first 24 hours but increases after that.

If you have ruptured membranes - broken waters - before you go into labour, you will be monitored closely for any sign of infection, including a change in the nature of the leaking fluid, a change in how you feel or any temperature that you have. You may have swabs taken and blood tests. In some cases the infection can spread in the placenta and there is a risk of it getting into the mothers blood stream. This is called chorioamnionitis and is usually an indication for delivering your baby as soon as possible. If things are alright, you will just be monitored, but you may be advised to take antibiotics as you go into labour.

Sometimes babies can acquire infections merely through travelling through the birth canal. A baby born by elective Caesarean section should not be prone to infections.

The bacterium that we are most concerned about is one that is called a Group B streptococcus. Group B strep or GBS for short. This germ can live quite happily in the birth canal without causing any disturbance to you. You can have it and may not know that it is there. To make things even more confusing it can come and go, so if we look for it, it can be there one minute and gone the next! Probably up to a third of all women will carry GBS at some stage.

Whilst it is essentially harmless in mothers, it can be very nasty in babies. If you have any history of having GBS in the past, you may well be offered antibiotics in labour. Otherwise we are likely to consider your baby at risk of developing GBS infection and treating accordingly.

As you can see we are really quite neurotic about the slightest chance that a baby might have an infection and we would normally consider the possibility in any baby that was out of sorts. This would include a baby with a temperature, one who was breathing fast, had jaundice, poor feeding seemed sleepy or many other reasons. If we suspect an infection we would normally perform some tests. These would usually include blood tests and urine tests. Sometimes other tests would be indicated including a chest X-ray and Lumbar Puncture (spinal tap).

A lumbar puncture is where some spinal fluid is taken off the spine to look for meningitis. Unfortunately babies with meningitis can present with very subtle signs and a lumbar puncture is the only way of knowing for sure if they do or don't have it. The information can be very important; clearly if a baby does have meningitis then they are going to need a different course of antibiotics. Babies tolerate lumbar punctures very well. There is always a lively debate amongst Paediatricians as to whether we are doing too many or too few lumbar punctures.

Once the tests are performed, the baby will be given antibiotics. These would usually be given intravenously via a drip. This is the best way of ensuring that the proper level of antibiotic enters the body.

Some test results will be available in a few hours. These preliminary results will point to whether a bacterial infection is present. If they are all clear, we need to wait for the final results, to make sure that everything is clear - these usually take at least 48 hours.

In the unlikely event of the results being positive, then the antibiotics may need to be changed and are probably going to be continued for somewhere between 5 days and 3 weeks - depending on the organism.

If the results are negative, then the antibiotics can be stopped sooner. In most cases this would be as soon as the 'all clear' is received from the labs, usually at 48 hours. However, for babies that have seemed particularly sick, we may want to carry the antibiotics on for a bit longer, usually about 5 days.

Are there any problems with antibiotics? There are a lot of misconceptions about antibiotics. Basically they are incredibly safe. It is essentially unheard of for babies to have allergies to antibiotics. Because they can affect normal helpful bacteria, they can cause short term problems like stomach upsets or thrush, but these resolve when the antibiotics are stopped. Antibiotics do not alter the immune system in any way. The idea that the immune system is weakened by antibiotics is a total myth.

GETTING HOME - THE FIRST FEW WEEKS

Growth & Feeding / Growth/centile charts:

When babies are weighed, they are plotted on growth charts. These sometimes cause some degree of confusion and anxiety. It is important to remember that:

- Growing is not a competition; you only compare yourself to yourself
- In any measurement, half of us are below average

The charts have lots of different lines across them - the centiles. These lines indicate how many babies you would expect to find below the line. For example at the 0.4th centile, 0.4 babies in 100 (or 4 in 1000) will be below the line, at the 50th centile 50% or half of all babies will be below that line and at the 99th centile, 99% of babies will be below it.

The charts are made by looking at large groups of people and measuring them at different ages. This will give us an idea of what is normal and what is unusual. The charts are very useful and to people that use them all the time are straightforward. They are more useful when they are used over a period of time - to see how your baby is growing, rather than for single measurements.

It does not matter what centile your baby is on, as long as they are healthy. In the UK with a population of about 50 million people, two hundred thousand of them will be below the 0.4th centile. And if all of these people grew by 2 feet, then they would be bigger, but because centiles measure the whole population, the next 200,000 shortest people, whatever their height, would be below the 0.4th centile. So the actual point on the line does not really matter.

It is true that babies that are born either extremely big or extremely small have an increased risk of having a medical problem and they may need to be investigated. Most of these babies however are normal.

Because the centile chart measures growth, we expect a baby to grow along their centile. This means that a baby who is on the 9th centile should continue to grow along it. Many people get concerned that their baby is 'below average weight'. I hope I have made it clear that this is a misplaced worry as long as they are growing as they should.

The other important point is that we normally plot a baby's growth calculating their age from when they were supposed to be born, rather than when they were actually born. If a baby is born two months prematurely then at six months of age, they should really only be four months old and should be plotted as being four months old.

Many seeming problems of growth are caused by 'mistakes'. If the weight, head size or age of the baby is either calculated wrongly or put on the wrong place on the chart, this can cause a lot of unnecessary concern.

There are a number of real situations in relation to centile that may cause concern:

- Moving down through the centiles: If a baby is born with weight on the 75th centile and over time his weight falls to the 50th, then 25th and then the 9th centile, then we would assume that the baby was failing to thrive - and not growing appropriately. At each of these times the baby's weight may be increasing, it is just not keeping up with what we would expect.

- The exception to this would be if a mother has poorly controlled diabetes in pregnancy. In this situation, the baby can be overfed in the womb and be born too large. Over the next few weeks, the baby will find its proper line. For example a baby girl born at 4.5kgs - Over 9lbs, will be at birth, above the 99th centile. It is possible that she was only meant to be 3.5kg (just over 7lb). If this was the case, we would expect her weight to fall to the 50th centile over the first few months, before stabilising.

- As well as weight, we also routinely measure the size of a baby's head - the head circumference. If this is falling through the centiles, the concern would be that the baby's brain may not be growing adequately.

- Moving up through the centiles: As far as a baby's weight is concerned this usually happens only if a baby has been struggling in the womb and is born too small, as may happen in a mother with raised blood pressure. In this situation we expect the baby to show 'catch up growth' in the first few months, before finding their correct line.

- Rarely, there are medical conditions which cause too rapid growth, but as said these are very uncommon.
- If a baby's head size is growing too quickly, the concern would be that there may be a build up of fluid on the brain (hydrocephalus) this would need urgent attention. In this situation, an ultrasound can usually quickly identify the diagnosis.

Growth in the first few weeks of life

Newborn babies will usually lose weight in the first few days of life. They should regain this weight over the next few days and then continue to grow. As with all general rules you will always find somebody to challenge them, but, the general rules about weight are:

- Weight loss of up to 10% of birth weight is normal in the first three days of life
- After this there should be some weight gain every day
- By 10 days of age a baby should weigh at least as much as she did when she was born
- Weight gain after this is about 7g/kg/day - or the old health visitors' formula of 'an ounce a day except for Sunday'
- Normal milk intake - before weaning is about 120-150ml/kg/day or 2 fl oz/lb/day

The figure for normal milk intake applies to babies once they have established feeding. This can take a few days to happen. So, in the first few days of life they will feed a bit less than this. If you are breast feeding, you may get some feeling of milk coming out, or see it happening. For a first timer feeder it is difficult to know if you have got things right until you know for sure that it is going right. Don't be afraid to ask for help and advice. In the first few days of life minimal milk requirements would be (more or less):

AGE	INTAKE ML/KG/DAY	INTAKE FL OZ/LB/DAY
0-24 hours	60	1
24-48 hours	90	1 ½
48-72 hours	120	2
72-96 hours	120-150	2- 2 ½

So, for example a baby weighing 3 kg, on the first day of life should drink 180 ml (3kg X 60 ml/kg/day) and if he feeds every four hours, he would get six feeds a day and need about 30 ml in each feed.

Using an empirical (pounds and ounces example) a 7 lb baby on the second day of life should drink 10 ½ fl Oz. (7lb X 1 ½ fl oz/lb/day)

If he was feeding every 4 hours, that is six feeds per day, he should have at least almost 2 fl oz per feed.

Weight loss of up to 10% of birth weight is normal in the first three days of life.

Weight alone should never be used to assess the wellbeing of a baby. If your baby is unwell, or doing things he shouldn't be doing or not doing the things that he should, he needs attention regardless of his weight.

For a number of reasons, at birth babies are born 'over hydrated' - that is, that they hold in extra water in their body. The most likely benefit for doing this is that it can take a few days for breast milk supply to be fully up and running. So, during the first few days of life, the baby may not be able to get with as much fluid as he would normally need, but is able to live on his stores. In the first 2-3 days of life, with these things going on, it is not unusual for the baby to lose some weight.

How much weight is it normal to lose?

The standard teaching is that babies may lose up to 10% of their birth weight. Like all accepted knowledge, you will find people who will argue that this is just an old wives tale and whilst they may be right, we also know that some old wives can tell some pretty good tales sometimes-and this is probably one of them.

So, let's accept that we expect your baby to lose some weight in the first 2 or 3 days. This is entirely normal and not a cause for concern. We will go with the general rule that this can be up to 10% or 1/10 of the birth weight.

We are going to do a bit of maths here. If you want to skip to the next section, go ahead. You are an expectant parent and you have better things to do than sums, we'll let you off. If you want to stay with us for this bit, hold on to your hats and let's go.

To do the calculations for this, it is much easier to use the metric system: I know that for most people mentioning kilograms and maths in the same sentence is enough to give you palpitations but, hold on and we will get through this together.

So a baby weighing 3.120 Kg at birth could be expected to lose 312g by day 3, giving him a weight of 2.808 Kg. If his weight is less than this you should get him checked out.

An easier way to think about this would be to know your babies birth weight in grams or kilograms and use the following formula.

My baby's weight should not fall below: **Birth weight x 0.9**

You can do this sum very easily- calculators are allowed and then when you weight your baby you only have to check if she is more or less than the 'danger weight'.

Using our above example, a baby born at 3.12kg should not drop their weight below 3.12 x 0.9 Kg = 2.808kg.

You could do the same using pounds and ounces, but first you have to convert the baby's weight to ounces only.

So, if your baby weighs 7lb 8oz, there are 16 ounces in a pound, so 7lb is 112 ozs (7x16), 7lb 8 oz is 120 oz and so your baby should not fall below

- in ounces - 120 X 0.9 = 108 = 6lb 12oz.

Given this information, if you have a reliable set of scales at home, you might want to weigh your baby yourself if you are worried about him.

It is true that if a baby is not well, then she may lose weight. So, if you are worried about your baby, please don't rely on a small change in weight alone to give you false reassurance.

Breast v. Bottle

As I sit down to write this section I can hear the cocking of rifles with people ready to shoot me down at every comma. So, before we start this section let me lay my colours to the mast.

Anybody who cares about children should contact, or better still join, Baby Milk Action, 34 Trumpington Street, Cambridge, CB2 1QY, UK.

Phone: 01223 464420 (www.babymilkaction.org)

This is a fantastic charity which fights against the peddling of formula feeds to the poor countries of the world.

Formula feeding is responsible to a great degree in over 1 million avoidable baby deaths per year in poor countries of the world. This is for 3 main reasons:

1. The water supply is unclean so the milk is made up with dirty water, which causes diarrhoea in the babies. This is a common cause of death.
2. Because the milk is so expensive, people can't afford to make it up properly so may use 1 scoop per bottle rather than 8 scoops per bottle. - This means that the babies are extremely malnourished.
3. Even when used like this, the amount they have to spend on milk can mean that there is not enough money to buy food for the rest of the family who suffer malnutrition.

I have no doubt that in these circumstances breast milk is, by over a million lives a year, the best option. I even try to boycott those companies that peddle formula milk in the poor countries and encourage others to do the same.

In rich countries things may be a little different. I know that breast is best, but don't know by how much it is best. There are certainly reports that breast fed babies have fewer ear infections and episodes of diarrhoea and vomiting in the first year of life and, perhaps some evidence, although that is disputed that they might gain a few IQ points.

Instinctively breast-feeding seems the right thing to do and I agree that mothers should be encouraged to breast-feed and we should delight rather than despair when they choose to do it in public.

However, I am also wary of the evangelical breast feeder. We have to be sensitive to the fact that breast-feeding just does not seem to work for some people. As we keep on saying, if you wanted to breast feed, but it hasn't worked you are likely to feel a complete failure. Unfortunately, the pervading culture can make you feel even worse.

In a rich country, like ours, the absolute benefits of breast-feeding are harder to establish. If it is not working for you, then you may have to use formula. **A baby will do better bottle feeding well from a contented mother than she will breast feeding badly from a distressed and depressed one.** Or, as I said much to the relief of one lady 'There's more to being a mother than just shoving your breast in its mouth every few hours'.

Unfortunately, we often have fairly inadequate breast-feeding support and mothers are just left alone with the assumption that 'because it's natural and right; it will just come naturally'. However, as they say 'For something that's meant to come naturally, it does take an awful lot of practice'.

An added pressure is that a mother is expected to be the sole breast feeder of her child. It is only in a 'Western' culture where one lady is expected to be the sole feeder of her child. In cultures where there is exclusive breast feeding, they have wet nurses that can feed a baby if a mother is unable to and sometimes women in a community will help each other out by feeding each others babies. Not only that, but our culture expects mothers to not only breast feed, but also to maintain most of their other functions as well.

Commonly, in the first few weeks, bottle fed babies put on weight more quickly than breast fed babies. As every woman measures her maternal worth by how well her baby feeds and how well her baby grows, this is a further challenge to breast feeders. If you are breast-feeding, then this may happen but as long as your baby is growing normally is not a cause for concern. Although many parents see their baby's growth as some kind of competition, a baby only needs to grow along the appropriate centile.

I think I am still alive so let's continue.

The most important thing is that your baby does feed properly. It is a little hard to know what this means, especially as babies may not feed brilliantly well over the first few days of life.

Also, a hungry baby will suck, even if he is not getting any milk and after sucking for some time he may be exhausted and go to sleep, which makes everyone feel that he has filled himself up. So, knowing if a baby is breast-feeding well is quite difficult to work out, especially for the first time mother.

Let's look at the 2 components of breast-feeding:

1. Are you producing enough milk?
2. Is your baby is taking enough milk from your breast?

Are you producing enough milk?

Milk production tends to increase in the first few days after delivery. It is largely driven by hormones and physical stimulation. It is important to appreciate the importance of physical stimulation in breast milk production, so that placing your baby to the breast, even if your milk has not come through is vital.

Remarkably, women who have adopted babies without ever being pregnant themselves have succeeded in breast-feeding their babies. In this situation, simply putting the baby to the breast has been enough to stimulate adequate breast milk production to exclusively breast-feed.

You will know when breast milk production has been properly established, because you will be aware of your breasts filling, they are also likely to leak some milk at various (or most) times of the day and you will get used to the feeling of being emptied. For the first timer it can be difficult to know if you are feeling the right things, so the more help and advice that you get; the better. As well as midwives, most hospitals will have specialist breast feeding advisers who can help. The NCT and LaLecheLeague are breast feeding support groups that also offer wonderful support.

Is your baby getting enough milk?

This can be a little more difficult to gauge. If you are producing milk and your baby is sucking for 15-30 minutes and then seems contented then the chances are that your baby is getting enough.

If your baby is not getting enough she may initially be unsettled and irritable, although this can progress through to drowsiness over a few days, giving the impression that she has become more settled and contented.

Unfortunately midwives do not do home visits as often as they used to and certainly don't weigh babies as often as they did twenty years ago. Because some of the breast-feeding 'promotion' makes them believe that breast-feeding has to work, they will sometimes not even acknowledge the possibility that it might fail. This means it can be quite hard to convince your midwife that there is a problem.

You might hear comments like 'It's your first baby', or 'carry on, let's give it a week or so'.

But, if there is a problem I would not be happy waiting a week. Babies can get dehydrated quite quickly, so any concern needs to be acted upon promptly.

The best way to assess feeding in a baby is by weighing the baby. As we suggested there is misplaced concern that weighing babies too often will make mothers stop breastfeeding. There is actually research to suggest that breastfeeding mothers are reassured by having their babies weighed every few days at the beginning.

As explained above, we expect a little bit of weight loss in the first few days, with a return to birth weight by about 10 days of age.

Breastfeeding on medication

So, here you are ready and waiting breasts filled with milk eagerly waiting to feed your baby. But, wait a minute you are on some medication and you are told that feeding whilst on medication may not be safe. You look at the medicine packet and it will probably advise you not to breast feed on this medication.

The reason for this is that drug companies do not like exposing themselves to any risks, so it is easiest for them to say 'don't breastfeed if you take our drugs'. Again things are not so simple.

Many drugs that will cross over into breast milk, but for most of these the amount present in the breast milk will be so small as to be barely noticeable and highly unlikely to have any effect on your baby.

For example, if you are taking anti depressants and are keen to breast feed. It is true that some of the drug will cross over into your milk, (you can find out exactly how much from your doctor.) But, we need to take the whole picture into account.

You should make sure that you need to be on medication and ensure that you are on the best one for you that gets into your milk as little as possible. Remember that your baby needs you to be as well as you possibly can be and not taking essential medication does you or your baby no favours whatsoever.

Also consider the benefits of breast feeding. If you will feel bad about not being allowed to feed, this can affect your well being, which is not good for you or your baby. Additionally, you have to balance whether breast milk plus a miniscule dose of a drug is better or worse than formula feeds.

Every doctor should have access to a drug handbook, such as the BNF (British National Formulary) which has realistic information about breast feeding whilst on medication. You can discuss this with your doctor and take a balanced view as to whether you want to feed or not.

If you really want to distress a mother tell her that her baby is not feeding. There seems to be a near universal need of mothers to feed their babies. Different ethnic groups might claim this as their own saying she is being a typical Jewish/Italian/Asian mother. But, in my experience all mothers are the same.

There is tremendous anxiety that your baby is not feeding, especially if he is also small, even if he is growing appropriately. There are limitless opportunities to undermine as regards feeding. Great examples are:

- I had 312 children and they all licked the plate clean and asked for more
- Maybe it's because you are too tense
- Perhaps it's how you make the food

Parents of children who are not great feeders can answer you back and you will never know if they are right. By saying:

- It's strange he eats much better when you are not around!

Overfeeding

Overfeeding is something that is much more likely to occur in bottle-fed, rather than breast fed babies and this is because bottle fed babies have access to a limitless supply of milk.

Sucking is a basic reflex. So, if you put anything in a baby's mouth it will suck. A breast has a limited supply of milk, so that although a baby may suck for half an hour or so, most of the milk is consumed in the first 10 minutes, with the rest being more about comfort and bonding than nutrition. It's a bit like guzzling away at the soup and main course and then spending a leisurely relaxing time picking at the after dinner mints.

If a baby is given a bottle, he will continue to suck and because there is a constant supply of milk, his stomach will fill and then overfill. He will be sucking because that is what babies do, rather than because he is hungry. You might say that 'his eyes are bigger than his stomach'. As his stomach becomes too full, the baby is likely to posset some of the milk. In babies with some degree of reflux, this is likely to be even more pronounced.

It is easy to over-estimate the quantity of vomit and believe that the baby has thrown up all of his feed. A parent's natural reaction to this is to replace the lost feed. The baby is then offered another bottle which, being a baby he will suck at. He will then take in even more milk on an already full stomach and is likely to throw up even more, generating further anxiety and causing more bottles to be produced and a vicious cycle to commence.

Although overfed babies can have very significant vomiting, the diagnosis is easily made because:

- The baby is growing appropriately, that is anything that is vomited out is purely surplus to the baby's requirements
- There is an excessive intake of milk

How much milk should a baby drink?

Metric
- A normal baby should consume 120-150 ml per Kg of milk per day
- So a 4 Kg baby would consume about 480-600 ml per day
- If the baby was having 6 bottles a day (feeding every 4 hours)

- One would expect each bottle to contain 80-100ml

Empirical
- A normal baby should consume
- 2-2½ fl oz per lb per day
- So a baby of 10 lbs should take 20-25 fl oz per day
- If the baby was having 6 bottles a day (feeding every 4 hours)
- One would expect each bottle to contain about 3- 4 fl oz

Clearly, if a baby is vomiting and overfeeding, the first thing to do is to try cutting down the feeds. It is always a little difficult to know what role reflux disease plays in all of this. Some babies with reflux disease find that some milk is soothing, so seem very hungry. Sometimes they seem hungry because they keep sucking their hands. They do this because saliva is alkali and can help to neutralise the acid in their stomach and oesophagus. So, they just look hungry and if a bottle is put into their mouths they will suck.

Essentially, as overfeeding makes reflux worse cutting down the feeds should be done first. Often this will reduce reflux symptoms, but if they persist they can be treated in the normal way.

How often should you feed?

This is another controversial area. In one corner you will have people telling you to demand feed, even if this means you are constantly feeding your baby, whilst in the other corner you will have the 'feed by the clock' brigade and tell you to use your watch rather than your baby's signals.

You've guessed it. They are both right. They are also both not quite right. As with all of this baby business it is useful to think of our basic goals:

- Your baby is receiving the correct amount of milk
- Your baby is content and happy
- You are as content and happy as possible

If your baby is growing along their centile, then they are almost certainly getting the correct amount of milk.

After the first few days, babies should be feeding every 3-5 hours. It is possible to train a baby to feed by the clock and if they are hungry before a feed you can try holding off by soothing them or just closing your ears. Essentially you should choose what works best for you and your family.

If they are permanently unsettled or take very small frequent feeds then they are quite likely to have reflux disease and this may need looking at.

Meconium and passing stool

The first stool that babies pass is called meconium. The word comes from the Greek for 'poppy juice' because that is what it looks like! It is a green/black tarry substance, which is made up largely of old cells from the lining of the bowel.

If babies are distressed before delivery, they may pass meconium whilst still in the womb (see below), but normally they will pass it in the first few days after birth. Once your baby has passed meconium it is essentially a signal that their bowels are almost certainly 'put together OK'.

The majority of babies will pass meconium within 48 hours of birth. If your baby has not passed meconium by this stage, you should discuss it with your midwife or doctor. Obviously they will need to check that the anus is present and patent. There is a rare condition called Hirschprung's disease which is caused by a problem with the nerve supply to the bowel and causes serious constipation. If left untreated it can cause other significant problems. If Hirschprung's is suspected then an operation will almost certainly be necessary, but the outcome is excellent.

Once your baby starts feeding he should start producing more normal stools. These are likely to be yellow or greenish and can appear a bit seedy. Old wives tales abound about how often a baby should 'go' and for every grandmother that tells you that breast fed babies don't poo very often there will be another who says that they poo after every feed. I am not aware of any study that has checked this out.

More importantly, it really doesn't matter how often they go, what matters is how they go. Pooing for babies should be easy and comfortable. You should have no idea when it is happening and your baby should be the same before, during and after a poo.

The Crying baby

Helpful advice for the unhelpful relative:

All babies cry - it's what they do, what do you expect if you have a baby? Whilst it is true that all babies cry, their crying is not always normal. Excessive crying in a baby is likely to indicate that they are in pain. Some painful conditions, such as heartburn (reflux) - can change with the way a baby is positioned. When they are very young it is probably over the top to claim that 'he knows when I am around and always wants to be picked up' it is more likely that when you pick him up, gravity helps keeps his stomach contents in his stomach. Similarly, the child who does not like being picked up is more likely to have a broken bone or infected joint - both of which will be more painful if they are moved, rather than being a 'loner'.

So, if your baby is crying excessively it is worth getting them checked out by a doctor or midwife. Sometimes the cause of crying can be hard to detect and if you (or more importantly your baby) still feel unhappy then you should ask again and ask somebody else if necessary.

Some of the causes of a crying baby include:

- Hunger - underfed
- Reflux Oesophagitis (heartburn)
- Constipation/stool withholding
- Cow's milk protein intolerance
- Gastroenteritis
- Ear Infection
- Oral Thrush
- Eczema
- Fractures - these can happen during delivery
- Joint swelling
- Cerebral irritation

And sometimes, whatever you do for them, there are some babies who just seem to cry.

But, crying normally means that a baby is in pain. Nobody likes to be in pain. I am amazed that there are still people who question whether babies 'really' feel pain - of course they do and, there is plenty of evidence to show that they remember pain and being in pain can have long term consequences. So, I believe it is essential to try and find out what is making a baby cry. If there is something that can make them cry less and be more comfortable then they should get this as soon as possible. If despite all of this they continue to cry, then at least we can say we did all that we could and your baby might just be one that cries.

A lot of causes of crying will get better by themselves over time - a few months or so. You may have well meaning relatives telling you that you screamed non-stop for a year and then stopped. That's fine, but please don't let it stop you getting help for your baby.

Of equal importance is the impact that a crying baby has on its parents. We all have our limits. If we have to listen to our baby crying nonstop it makes us feel helpless and tired and frustrated and thousands of other difficult feelings that we did not sign up to when we wanted to be parents. As a parent you are probably completely exhausted. If your baby is crying excessively you will not only be worried about your baby but also worn out yourself. When you are this shattered it can be hard to function properly. It is certainly hard to be as patient and nice as you would like to be. You should not feel bad about this. Giving yourself a break is important. Do not underestimate how important it is for your baby that you are as healthy, relaxed and happy as you possibly can be.

It is important to:

- Share the load - as long as there is somebody with the baby, you can leave to get a bit of calm
- Accept any help when it is offered
- Ask for help if you need it. Everybody needs some time out. You are not a failure if you need a break to catch up on sleep or have an uninterrupted bath. Try to find people that are happy to help

If you need to talk to somebody urgently you can call Cry-sis 08451 228 669 (7 days a week - 9am - 10pm) or Parentline plus www.parentlineplus. org.uk

They have a 24/7 free helpline 0808 800 2222

You might need to speak to your GP or health visitor. If you are feeling low or depressed, a baby crying can make things worse, which in turn can make you more sensitive to the crying. Your GP and health visitor will see many people with similar problems.

Hearing your baby cry is hard. Unfortunately, crying babies are more likely to be 'abused'. This is often simply because parents 'lose it'. If you feel that you are heading towards this, you must let somebody know.

Colic

A lot of baby crying is related to 'stomach' problems. These may be loosely called Colic. However, this is not a very helpful word, largely because if we say that a baby has colic, we often don't look very hard at trying to make them better.

Whilst it is true that a number of babies with symptoms will improve over 3-6 months, quite a few do not. Also, if treated properly they can get better much quicker. Unfortunately the standard over-the-counter colic drops usually make no difference. There is no evidence that homeopathic remedies or cranial osteopathy make any difference either.

Most of the time a change of baby milk does not help - indeed most milks are essentially the same with the main difference between them being the name or label. The main treatable causes of crying are gastro-oesophageal-reflux, constipation and milk intolerance.

There does seem to be a type of crying which is limited to a few hours every day, usually in the afternoon or evening. At all other times the baby seems completely content, but just has these bad few hours. This usually gets better after a few months and is often called 'three month colic'. If the crying is more persistent or there is a possible cause then you should not have to wait for three months before dealing with it.

Gastro-oesophageal Reflux

Gastro-oesophageal reflux or heartburn is very common in babies - in fact most babies have it to some degree. It is caused by regurgitation of stomach contents. As these are usually acidic, the acid can damage the lining of the oesophagus (gullet) which makes it sensitive and painful.

A common misconception is that a baby that does not vomit can not have reflux. This is not true; the stomach contents can go half way up and still cause pain without necessarily causing vomiting. However, we can be too quick to diagnose reflux and often say that any baby that vomits has it. Essentially we only need to worry about it if it is worrying your baby. If your baby is being sick, but is not bothered by it, then no real treatment is necessary, but do make sure that your baby is not being overfed.

Classic symptoms of reflux are:

- **Crying:** Often dependent on position. Because gravity can help prevent reflux, babies will often prefer to be upright. They are usually in this position when being held and you may think that they need to be held all the time. They will tend to be more uncomfortable when lying down - such as during nappy changes and will often be difficult to get to sleep and wake in pain every few hours.
- **Posturing:** The pain will sometimes make babies wriggle, arch their backs and turn their head to the left. These strange movements and positions are known as posturing.
- **Vomiting/possetting:** Pretty obvious!
- **Poor feeding:** If feeding is associated with pain, babies may take limited amounts of food.
- **Putting things in their mouths:** As we have said above the saliva helps neutralise the acid. By putting their hands in their mouths this can be misinterpreted as hunger.

Treatment

There are some tests for reflux, but these are usually unpleasant and invasive. Normally the first test is to see if your baby gets better with treatment. The type of treatment will depend on your baby's symptoms.

Mechanical:

Keep your baby upright as much as possible - day and night.

Feeding:

Reduce feed volumes. As mentioned above, babies should drink about 120-150 ml of milk per day for each kg of body weight. This is about 2fl oz of milk per pound of weight per day. If your baby is overfeeding this will certainly make vomiting and reflux worse.

Thicken feeds - with either a feed thickener or using one of the Anti-reflux or Stay-Down milks. The stay-down milks harden in the stomach by reacting with acid in the stomach. So, they will not work if your baby is using acid reducing drugs.

Medication:

Although it is hard to stop reflux, a number of drugs are used to treat the symptoms.

Alginates:

E.g. Gaviscon. These work by thickening the stomach contents making it more difficult to 'reflux'. The drug might also stop acid coming into contact with the lining of the oesophagus.

They may help mild reflux, but can be difficult to give if you are breastfeeding and can cause constipation.

Reducing acid secretion:

These drugs reduce the amount of acid produced by the stomach, so that any 'reflux' is not painful. They are often highly successful. Examples are Ranitidine, Omeprazole and Lansoprazole. These drugs all appear to be very safe.

Motility stimulants:

E.g. Domperidone - these work by strengthening the muscles between the oesophagus and stomach and also by making the stomach empty more quickly. This class of drugs may not work as well in small babies as they do in older children and adults.

Symptoms of reflux tend to improve over the first year of life - as the stomach muscles mature, the diet becomes more solid and the child spends more time upright. In some children symptoms can continue for longer and we know that older children and adults can also suffer from it. Some children with untreated reflux can become a bit difficult to feed later on, probably because they associate eating with pain. They can also be babies who easily vomit.

Constipation/Stool withholding

This can happen at any age. If pooing hurts - for example if your baby gets a bit constipated, they may not want to poo again. This will lead to holding the poo in. There will be a battle between their bowels wanting to poo and their bottoms and brains wanting to hold on. This struggle can be painful.

If they are successful at stopping the poo coming, you might not be aware of what has been going on.

Symptoms

Crying:

This can continue for long periods of time. Often a baby can seem inconsolable.

Altered stool:

This does not always happen and if you are first time parents you may not know what normal baby stool looks like.

Being unsettled:

A lot of the wriggling and back arching that we mentioned in a refluxing baby can happen in stool withholding too.

Painful pooing/ being more settled after a poo:

If your baby is calmer after going for a poo, it is likely that this is what has been bothering him. However, if he has only done 'yesterday's poo' and still has 'today's poo' inside, he can still seem unsettled.

Treatment

The mainstay of treatment is to get your baby doing soft easy poos. The right treatment is the one that works. Useful things to try include:

- Offering extra water (120-180ml 0r - 4-6 fl oz per day) there is little benefit in adding sugar
- Consider orange juice/ prune juice or pureed pears
- Laxatives - e.g. Lactulose. The right dose being the one that works

Once your baby is pooing we need to keep on going until their bowel habit returns to normal- and this may take some time.

Cow's Milk Protein Intolerance (CMPI)

In some babies the underlying problem is CMPI - which should not be confused with lactose intolerance (Lactose is a milk sugar and an intolerance usually causes diarrhoea). There is growing evidence that a number of crying babies have CMPI. Indeed as symptoms of CMPI include reflux and altered bowel habit it is often worth thinking about this.

Again the only real test is to try a cow's milk protein free diet. Unfortunately, cow's milk protein (CMP) can get into breast milk, so a breastfeeding mother may need to try a dairy free diet.

If you are using formula, there are a few changes to consider. Some of the easy digest or comfort milks are partially hydrolysed and seem to be effective if the symptoms are mild. In children over 6 months it may be worth trying a soya based formula. Soya milks are not generally recommended in children under 6 months of age and a small number of children who react to Cows Milk Protein also react to soya protein.

The next step would be trying 'hydrolysed' milk. These are highly processed milks - which are usually only available on prescription.

Unfortunately they often don't taste great, but babies usually get used to them quite quickly. If a CMP free diet is going to work, it should become evident in the first few weeks.

If your baby improves on one of these milks, it is hard to know whether the improvement is caused by the change of milk or whether this is just a coincidence. The only way of knowing is by offering your baby their old formula. So, normally after a few weeks on the new formula they will be challenged with the old one, to see if it really was a milk problem. If it is not then we can restart the ice cream and pizzas!

If your baby does have CMPI they often grow out of it by a year or so of age.

Sleep

Advice for interfering relatives or friends:

∇ Remember: exhaustion is likely to make the parents more amenable to any advice you give.
∇ They will appreciate you chuckling and reminding them of how they used to sleep in late at weekends and how this is now payback time. They will be delighted to hear that you may be getting lots of sleep - just knowing that will make them feel better.
∇ Under no circumstances should you offer to look after their baby whilst they sleep, as this will completely undermine them as parents and may be the 'last straw'.

As a new parent this is something which you will remember doing in the past and crave doing again. There is little to compare with the exhaustion of childbirth and parenthood.

In many Primitive societies a mother after giving birth is not allowed out for six weeks, relatives will look after her and provide her with meals; the extended family will look after the rest of her family. If she cannot feed her baby, then a wet nurse will do it for her.

Compare this to the advanced society that we are privileged to live in.

Here seconds after delivering a baby, a woman is sent home with little or no aftercare. Because we view birth as a natural event, we treat it as little more than a hard but rewarding 'day at the office'. The mother is expected to be up and running immediately.

In reality childbirth is more like running a marathon in the heat wearing a monkey costume. Leaving aside all the emotions, you are likely to be knackered afterwards. It is essential that you get as much rest as you possibly can. You should spurn no reasonable offer of help in the first few weeks and any spare moment can usefully be spent asleep.

One of the recurring themes in this book is to consider you all as part of a family. This means that you are not simply your baby's slaves. It is impossible to overemphasize the importance of parents feeling as good as they possibly can.

If you are exhausted at all times, it will affect your parenting ability and resilience. This can have a significant adverse effect on your baby's development. You also need to think about the impact that undue exhaustion will have on other children and on your relationship with your partner. If these suffer it is bad news for everybody - baby included.

There are likely to be times when you are just so exhausted that you need to sleep. This is normal. At these times somebody might offer to feed your baby whilst you sleep. In the absence of wet nurses this means giving your baby a bottle. If you are breast feeding this could be with your expressed milk, or with formula. I have never been greatly convinced about 'nipple confusion' babies seem to just get on with it.

As we have said many times, you have to look at the whole picture. Giving your baby a feed that you don't really want is better than giving him a mother that nobody really wants.

Newborn babies can sleep for 12-20 hours per day. They will tend to wake for feeds and settle quickly. Over the first few months they will have more time awake and will use this time for social interaction and exploration. They will normally last between three and five hours between feeds. By 6-8 weeks they do not really need a night feed, but might still want one.

Sleep is essentially a 'habit'. If we learn bad habits they can stick and the longer we don't change them, the more ingrained they become. So, the longer a baby is used to waking at night for a bottle and a cuddle, the more this habit will be established. Although a few babies seem to develop a good routine by themselves, most of them need some help.

An important skill for a baby to learn is how to get to sleep independently. Waking up at night is normal, even a few times. If you always attend to your baby the moment they wake up and then rock them to sleep, they will come to expect this every time that they wake. You can train your baby to go back to sleep by themselves.

In the first few weeks you should:

- Distinguish between day and night. Our brains produce hormones at night time which make the body realise that it is time for sleeping. Light can interfere with this. So, it is good not to have lights on too brightly at night and if you do need to get up, use dimmed lights or night lights as much as possible.
- Don't let your baby fall asleep in your arms. If she is used to feeling your body when she falls asleep she will come to expect this. Whilst this gives you a wonderful feeling now, you may live to regret it.
- Don't feed immediately. If you feed your baby the second that she wakes, she will associate waking with feeding, if you wait awhile, calm her, change her nappy etc then she will not expect a feed with every waking.

These three simple steps are said to double the chances of a baby sleeping through the night at three months of age. They basically teach your baby to go back to sleep again by themselves.

If your baby is very unsettled and waking frequently it is important to consider whether they are waking in pain.

Common causes would include:

- Reflux/ heartburn/Oesophagitis
- Constipation / stool withholding
- Colic

Less common causes are:

- Ear pain
- Bone/joint pain

- Muscle spasm
- Medication

It is important to rule these out, because the bottom line is that normally the only way to get a baby to sleep is by letting them scream. There really is no Plan B.

Obviously, if your baby is waking due to heartburn pain then letting them scream is pointless and cruel to them. If they are waking out of habit, not letting them scream is probably just cruel to you. You also have to remember that the longer you leave it, the more screaming there will be.

The simple way is really just to let her scream. There are some modifications to this - so-called extinction techniques. Here, you let her cry for a short period, then go in and settle her in as simple a way as possible. You then leave and let her cry for a bit longer and repeat this until she is back to sleep. This is often called 'controlled crying' and the time between your visits usually starts at a few minutes and extends to thirty minutes or even more.

The great advantage of controlled crying is that it makes you believe that rather than being mean and nasty, you are following a proper process. It is also very hard to hear your baby cry and not do anything about it. Controlled crying can make this feel easier. Ultimately 'letting her scream' and 'controlled crying' are equally effective.

The problem with both of them is that they are especially hard to carry out if you are exhausted. If you are barely sleeping and your baby wakes up, it is easy just to give them what they want; so that they will go back to sleep and you can steal another hour of bliss before the day starts. To let them scream which will steal that precious hour from you can be simply too much.

Often before you can start a behavioural sleep programme, you need to be as awake as possible. This could mean doing it at a time when there are people who can help. For example, I have known families where they have run shifts. One person has slept at relatives at night, whilst the other deals with the screaming. In the daytime the well-rested partner can let the tired one sleep.

In slightly older children a short course of medication can help. Occasionally that would be enough to break a habit, but most importantly, whilst the child is on medication you can get some sleep, which will give you some energy to enter into the 'behavioural battle'.

Unfortunately, a common problem is 'maternal martyrdom'. In this condition, the mother tries to protect everybody around her. For example if a baby stirs at night, the mother will rush to it. This is partly a maternal instinct, worrying about her newborn baby and partly wanting to protect the other people in the house. She doesn't want a crying baby to wake the other children or, worst of all, the child's father. As a consequence we see a family that is well rested and refreshed apart from a bedraggled, exhausted mother who can barely function. I often point out, that presumably the father was not overly interested in sleeping at the time of conception, so can be reasonably expected to lose some sleep afterwards.

Sibling Rivalry

I suspect that if you are reading this book you are probably a first time parent. By the time you are on to your second pregnancy, or even more, you will already know it all and won't be bothered with stupid books. So, unless you are expecting twins, triplets or more, you might think that this does not apply to you.

So, I will be brief. Sibling rivalry is as old as the bible. In fact the first pair of brothers in the bible had so many problems that one (Cain) killed the other one (Hevel or Abel). So if you have problems they are probably not as bad as Adam's and Eve's.

Most sibling rivalry is based on jealousy and the basic theory is that 'you love him more than you love me and I am going to give you a test to prove it'. So, your children will put you in difficult situations where you have to choose one over the other: it's my turn, he started it, he hurt me and you never tell him off. Basically you don't stand a chance.

Now, think about your oldest child. From birth they are the apple of your eye. If they are the first grandchild as well they can easily become the centre of the family's universe. Every movement word and achievement will be feted throughout the family.

Then you go and spring a sibling on them. They go from being everything to nothing. It's the baby this and the baby that and any morsel of time that you spend with your now neglected firstborn is very fragile. Any squeak from the new impostor and you stop in your tracks because 'the baby is crying'. For number one, it feels like he is only getting the scraps of your time and not only that, but in the few seconds that he might have your now divided attention you are less focussed and less fun than you used to be. Not surprising that he may get upset.

He also always seems to get the blame and is expected to be responsible, know better and share his things, because his rival is only a baby and does not know any better.

Yeah, really. I see it everyday in clinic how good a younger child is at stealing attention. You are coming to clinic to talk about your firstborn. Number two, has to come along, because you can't leave him anywhere else and he's normally not much trouble. You will be amazed that as soon as you enter my room, number two will cry/be hungry/ take my room apart/sit on your lap and pull your hair or sit on my lap and pull my beard. Anything in fact to make you remember who is boss. I bet you will fall for the trap. You will be indulgent of your little one. The older child will be asked to sit still/be patient or give his younger sibling a favourite toy in order to pacify him and allow the consultation to continue. In my experience as an observer, in life I was child two, is that the firstborn gets told off at least 10 times as often as a second born child.

There are some things that you can do to try and reduce this. Firstly, you must remember that older children may not be as excited as you will be at the prospect of the family size increasing. It is important that not everything becomes referenced to the new baby. Visiting relatives should appear at least as interested in the firstborn's new shoes as they are in his new sibling.

As they get older, it can be very useful to institute a rota system, which works best if it is easy to monitor. As we said before, the arguments are all to prove how unfair you are. If you decide that you are going to divide some things completely equally, they will find an area that you have not considered to challenge you. Taking turns to be in charge of the day can reduce arguments dramatically.

On a calendar, put the children's names on consecutive days. Whoever is in charge on that day can make all the important decisions, such as should we go to the park or swimming, cbeebies or CITV, peas or beans. This way they realise that there is no obvious favouritism. Ideally they also realise that they might as well be nice to each other, because tomorrow the boot will be on the other foot.

It is also wonderful to give each child some individual 'golden' time when they have your undivided attention. If time is very pressing, this can be linked to being in charge of the day. It is essential that at golden time, the other children are around but doing something else. The whole idea of it is that 'you are special too'. Spending time with the older child when the younger one has already gone to bed can defeat the purpose and makes it seem again that he only gets you when his younger sibling is not around.

NEWBORN SCREENING TESTS

Neonatal screening tests are part of the 'quality control' process that babies go through in the first few weeks of life. We have already discussed the newborn examination, which is essentially a way of checking to make sure that there are no obvious problems. This examination is repeated about six weeks later, usually by your GP. Partly because some conditions only develop after a few weeks and partly to make sure that nothing has slipped through the net from the first examination.

As well as the physical examination, your baby will be tested to see if they have a number of medical conditions. There are a number of considerations when deciding which medical conditions should be tested for.

- The test must be easy to do and it should be reliable
- The condition should be one where an early diagnosis will alter the outcome - that is the sooner it is known about the better
- There should be some treatment available that will change the outcome

A further consideration is how frequent a medical condition happens in a population. Testing for a condition that might arise once in a hundred years is simply not worth it.

All babies in the UK are screened for a number of different conditions. Most of these will be tested for with a blood spot test, taken by your midwife from your baby's heel, after your baby is a few days old. These are often referred to as the Guthrie test, although strictly, the Guthrie test is only one part of it. If any of the results are positive you will be informed in the next few weeks. If everything is clear, you should get the results back in 6-8 weeks.

A screening test does not confirm a diagnosis. If the results are positive, more tests will need to be performed to make sure either way.

The conditions that are screened for in the UK include the following. Some areas may also do other tests, your midwife or GP should be able to tell you about these.

- Hypothyroidism - an underactive thyroid affects about 1 in 4,000 babies. If this is untreated it can cause long term developmental problems. Treatment is simple - with thyroid replacement as a medicine. The earlier treatment starts the better.

- Phenylketonuria (PKU) In this condition, which affects about 1 baby in 10,000, an enzyme that is important in the breakdown of proteins is absent, more particularly the enzyme involved in breaking down the amino acid - phenylalanine. This means that there is a build up of Phenylalanine. At high levels this can be quite toxic and cause brain damage. If it is detected early then damage can be prevented by avoiding phenylalanine in the diet.

- Cystic Fibrosis. This affects about 1 in 2500 babies born in the UK. It is the most common genetic disease in the UK, with rates varying between ethnic groups. It causes problems in many different parts of the body - especially affecting the lungs and digestion. The earlier the condition is discovered, the sooner treatment can start. This is usually a combination of chest physiotherapy, nutritional support and prompt treatment of infections. The hope is that if it is detected very early; we can prevent or significantly slow down the damage that it causes. Unlike most genetic disease which are caused by a problem in only one gene, it seems that Cystic Fibrosis can happen due to any one of hundreds of different gene problems. This makes testing for it in babies a bit tricky. The current screening programme identifies about 97% of cases by looking at the most common gene problems. It is most sensitive for picking up babies of European origin. Babies with cystic fibrosis whose parents are not of European origin are more likely to have much rarer genetic changes which are more difficult to detect.

- If there is concern that a baby may have Cystic fibrosis, then there are other tests that can be conducted. Haemaglobinopathy: This is to test for haemoglobin abnormalities - especially sickle cell disease. Sickle cell disease makes abnormal adult haemoglobin which causes the red blood cells to break more easily. It is a very serious disease which has significant morbidity (causes illness) and mortality (can cause death) It is a problem essentially that occurs in children of Afro-Caribbean descent.

- Babies in the womb need to take their oxygen from the mother, so need a very 'greedy' haemoglobin - the foetal type. After birth this is no longer necessary and as the red blood cells are replaced they contain more 'adult' haemoglobin, so that by six months of age most of the haemoglobin is 'adult'.

The abnormal haemoglobin makes the red blood cells more fragile and this can cause a number of very serious problems. Before screening was widely used, the first presentation of a baby with sickle cell disease may have been with a life threatening illness. Early detection allows families to know about the condition and to start treatments that make serious problems very much less likely.

- Medium Chain Acyl Dehydrogenase Deficiency (MCADD): Is a long name for a condition affecting 1 in 10 000 children. In this condition babies have difficulty releasing stored energy. When we are ill, or fasting, as our sugar levels fall, we mobilise our stored energy to keep our bodies going. If we can't release the energy form its stores then the body can 'run out of fuel' this can be devastating. If the condition is diagnosed it is managed by making sure that the baby receives appropriate feeds frequently, especially at times when they may need extra energy - for example during an infection.

Further information can be found at the UK Newborn Screening Programme Centre: www.newbornbloodspot.screening.nhs.uk

- Hearing Loss: Approximately 1 baby in 500 will have hearing problems from birth. If this is identified and treated early then the outcome in relation to language and communication is much improved. Because it is often hard to be sure or not if your baby hears, all babies will have a hearing test in the first few weeks of life.

The test is painless; a little probe is placed in your baby's ear. The probe sends out clicks, if hearing is normal the ear will send back an 'echo' to the probe.

Sometimes, for example if your baby is a bit unsettled, the test may be inconclusive and may need repeating, if there is uncertainty, a slightly more complicated (but just as painless) test can be performed.

You will receive the results immediately. If there is a problem then you will be immediately referred to a hearing specialist.

The UK National Screening Portal www.screening.nhs.uk/newbornhearing-england offers more information.

Immunisations

It is remarkable how much of my life as a doctor is taken up participating in groups which conspire to line our own pockets whilst exposing innocent children to danger. My diary is jam packed with meetings that will forcibly remove children from families or pump them full of dangerous drugs. The most fun that we have is at the immunisation groups. Here we are paid ridiculous sums of money to inject children with toxins that will at best destroy their immune system and at worst destroy the child or even the entire planet!

If only life was like that. I don't recall ever receiving a penny from the vaccine manufacturers, but still maintain that vaccination is one of the biggest miracles of modern medicine. One of its problems is that it is so successful that we do not realise what it is protecting us against. Gone are the days of living in fear of polio. But it killed thousands and left many more with permanent handicap.

Similarly concerning pertussis (whooping cough) whilst many people remember it as a bad cough, in some children it caused brain damage or even death. Today, many babies who are admitted seriously ill to paediatric intensive care units have evidence of pertussis infection - because they are not yet immunised.

Other immunisations, such as Hib - have eradicated a whole host of horrible diseases. Conditions such as Epiglottitis, which would effectively cause 'internal strangulation', have, thankfully, become diseases of history. The meningococcus vaccine has caused a massive decline in the incidence of meningitis.

I have had the misfortune/ benefit of seeing most of the disease that we can prevent. I had my children vaccinated against everything.

There is a strong anti-vaccine lobby. Interestingly, whilst they say they are heroic campaigners revealing another conspiracy, this may not always be the case. The most recent anti vaccine group successfully discredited MMR for a while. This led to many extra cases and deaths. The main 'investigator' it transpired, was in the pay of lawyers who were fighting the vaccine manufacturers. He received hundreds of thousands of pounds to produce bogus research.

On the coat tails of his 'research', many clinics sprung up offering so-called single vaccines. These vaccines were not only less effective but also less safe than the combined MMR. It did not stop the marketing and clinics were making millions.

Which immunisations are given at what age varies across the world. It is influenced by many factors including which diseases are prevalent. For example many countries have routine immunisation against Hepatitis B or TB. In the UK these are only given to babies who are thought to be at highest risk.

The aim of vaccination is to protect your child as well and as soon as possible. Babies will make a better response the later they receive a vaccination, but this has to be balanced by the fact that they remain vulnerable until they receive it. Most vaccinations need booster doses to make sure that the immune system makes a strong sustained response.

Ideally it would be good to put all the vaccines in one injection. Unfortunately, some of the vaccines would react with each other so this is not always possible.

Sometimes people worry about 'antigen overload:' an antigen is a foreign substance - like a virus - that triggers the body to try to fight it off by mounting an immune response. In reality newborn babies meet thousands of different antigens everyday. The five or six they meet in a vaccine are neither here nor there.

All vaccinations can have side effects. These are usually mild and certainly less severe than the disease, which they are protecting against. After any immunisation a baby may become miserable and have a fever. More serious reactions are extremely rare. There is a little bit of evidence that giving paracetamol may make a vaccine less effective, but if your child is miserable, you can give them some.

In order to work, a vaccination has to stimulate the immune system to make antibodies so that if the real infection enters the body, your baby will be able to fight it off quickly before the disease can take hold - 'know your enemy'. Every invader looks different. The trick is getting the immune system to recognise them.

Ideally presenting the immune system with a small part of the germ can do this. This can often be enough for the immune system to produce a response. It is a bit like agreeing to meet a stranger. You can just describe some special signal that you will give so that they will recognise you, rather than describing yourself in detail. Clearly, there is a good chance that you will be recognised, but some chance that you will not. Similarly, the immune response made from these vaccines may be limited, but may be more than good enough. On the positive side, there is only a tiny risk of any side effects.

The next level would be where the immune system needs more information - in which case it may need to see the whole antigen. The antigen could be killed and therefore inactive. Using our analogy this is like sending the stranger a picture so that they will recognise you. Again, the immune response generated will be better than in the first case, but there is a slightly higher risk of side effects.

A final level is where the immune system needs a live infection to work. In this case the infection is usually 'disarmed' a bit, known as attenuated. In this situation it's like sending the stranger a picture, video, your bank details and inside leg measurements! A live germ is used, so this will cause an illness, usually the germ is so weak that you might not even know that it has happened. For example, it is quite common to have a bit of a rash a week or so after MMR.

Ideally we would like all vaccines to be like the first type, but which type of vaccine is used, depends on how good they are at getting a response and how serious the threat of the illness is. For example, the Oral (live) polio vaccine is much more effective at protecting against polio than the Inactivated (dead) one. The downside is that in one in a million or so cases the live one can actually cause a form of polio.

When there was lots of polio around it was best to make sure that everyone was well protected and although the vaccine may have caused one or two cases, it prevented many thousands of others. The balance has now changed and with polio being much rarer it is better to use the killed vaccine.

Obviously you can only catch an actual disease from a live vaccine and there are no reported cases of any of the live vaccines that we use today causing any problems. Indeed vaccines are changing all the time, with safer and more effective ones being produced.

Immunisation schedules vary across the world. We will examine the UK schedule. If you live overseas or travel overseas your baby may need to receive extra vaccinations.

Other vaccines are not routinely available in the UK but maybe available through your GP or specialist immunisation clinics. This includes immunisations against Hepatitis B – although this is offered to 'high risk' groups- and Chicken Pox (Varicella Zoster).

Age	Which Vaccines	Comment
2 months	2 vaccines DTaP/IPV/Hib (5-in-1) (first dose)	**Diphtheria** - a nasty disease that can cause the back of the throat to block up and lead to death. Tetanus - Can cause paralysis which can spread up the body- causing respiratory paralysis. The vaccine is made from a toxoid- the neutralised form of the toxin or poison that the germ releases **Acellular Pertussis** - Whooping cough is not only unpleasant but can have serious/ fatal complications. The vaccine comprises neutralised toxin and may contain other bits of the germ, which may stimulate the immune system, but will not produce an infection. It is possible that this new vaccine, whilst safer, does not provide the same amount of protection as the older vaccines, so more doses may be required. **Inactivated Polio** - Polio again can cause serious paralysis. Happily it is more or less eradicated from the world. The vaccine contains the killed germ. **Haemophilus Influenza b** - This bacterium was responsible for many serious infections including: meningitis, pneumonia and Epiglottitis. The vaccine contains part of the bacterium- so it will encourage an immune response without causing the disease.
	Pneumococcus - (first dose)	**Pneumocoocus** - This can cause very serious infections including pneumonia and meningitis. There are many different strains of the bacterium the vaccine covers the most common ones, it contains parts of the bacterial wall- to produce an immune response without giving an infection.
	Rotavirus 1st dose	Rotavirus is the major infection causing diarrhoea and vomiting in babies. It is a common cause of young babies coming to hospital with serious dehydration needing intravenous fluids. Because globally rotavirus is responsible for millions of infant deaths a year – especially in poor countries- the hunt for a safe effective vaccine has been going on for decades. It is very exciting that this new vaccine, which has been extensively tested does seem to fit the bill and is being introduced to the UK in 2013. It is a live attenuated (weakened) form of the virus and given as drops.

3 Months	5-in-1 (second dose) DTaP/IPV/Hib	
	Meningococcus C (first dose)	**Meningococcus C** - This is the bacterium that causes the classic, feared meningitis. At present vaccines for other strains of meningococcus are not very effective. So although the rate of meningococcal disease has been massively reduced since the vaccine was introduced, cases due to other strains can still occur. The vaccine again uses parts of the bacterial wall to generate an immune response, but cannot cause the disease.
	Rotavirus 2nd dose	
4 months	5-in-1 (third dose) DTaP/IPV/Hib	
	Pneumococcal (second dose)	
	Meningitis C (second dose)	
1 year	Hib (fourth dose) Meningitis C (third dose) Given as one vaccine Hib/MenC	
	Pneumococcal vaccine (third dose)	
	MMR (first dose)	**Measles/Mumps/Rubella** - this is a live attenuated vaccine, so there can be a very mild illness a week or two later. Although many people remember these as mild illnesses, they can actually be serious or even fatal. The concern with rubella is mainly to protect unborn babies. Anybody who is or will in future become a parent should make sure that they are protected against rubella.
3 ½ years (pre-school booster)	MMR (second dose)	
	DTaP/IPV (fourth dose	

There are very few genuine reasons why children should not have immunisations. The main one would be if there has been a very serious reaction to a previous one. Egg allergy does not appear to be a good reason to prevent immunising a child - even the MMR. If you are very worried, you should be able to have the vaccination done in hospital.

If your child is unwell at the time of immunisation you may want to delay it until they are feeling a bit better. The main reason for this is that the immunisation may make them feel a bit worse. If the immunisations are being continuously delayed, you might just want to bite the bullet and get them done. It really is important to get your children protected against these serious infections.

THE BITS YOU WOULD RATHER NOT HAVE TO READ

This section is aimed at giving you information which, I hope, you will not have reason to need. Although the vast majority of babies deliver without any trouble, a few do have problems. Even in this category, for the overwhelming majority, these problems are nothing more than a minor 'technical hitch' with no long term implications. Only a very small number of babies will have unanticipated problems which have a lasting legacy.

We will focus on some of the common problems that are seen in babies and discuss them in general terms. Clearly, every situation is different and it is important that you establish good communication with the team that are looking after your baby.

Communicating in hospital

Hospitals are interesting places. For those of us that work in them they are warm friendly and comfortable, whilst for people who use them they are cold, daunting and scary. Although those of us who live in them like to pretend that we are committed to making you feel welcome, we then tell you all the times that you can't come, what you can't do when you get here and who can't talk to you at the moment. Because we like coming to hospital to work, we can easily lose sight of how frightening it is to come as a patient.

We also develop our own language. We use complicated technical words, when simple ones would do and above all we love making abbreviations or acronyms, which act as a kind of secret language. So you may go from the DAU to the ANW then to the DS before going to the PNW and then home - not forgetting your TTAs. In normal language this is going to the clinic or Day Assessment Unit, then to the Antenatal Ward, Delivery Suite, Postnatal Ward and finally home - with any drugs you might need - your medication 'To Take Away'.

Trying to get any information out of this system is hard. To make things even more complicated, it is likely that you will meet a number of doctors, midwives, nurses and health care professionals (HCPs for short!) during your stay. There are a number of communication difficulties which commonly arise because of this.

- Nobody tells you anything, which is still, unfortunately all too common. Included in this category is being told things that you cannot understand, usually because too much jargon is being used.
- Different people tell you more or less the same thing but differently enough to get you completely confused. This really happens all the time. Also, any difference is likely to be of no significance, such as should you have 4 or 5 days of antibiotics.
- Different people tell you completely different things. This is very difficult. Somebody might tell you that you don't need an operation and another person might tell you that you need one now. Sometimes this happens because there is new information which the first person did not have. Or sometimes it just reflects that people do things differently and there is often no single correct answer as to how to manage a patient. 'There is more than one way to skin a cat'. But, it does make things bewildering.

In order to overcome this, some useful suggestions are:

- Write down any questions that you might have and answers that you are given. Although as doctors we like to see ourselves as invincible and infallible, we do rarely have a few chinks in our armour. It is not always possible to know what you are thinking. It is always helpful if we ask you, 'so what is it that you are really worried about?' But if we forget to do that, please tell us. For example, I often see children with minor niggles who are clearly fine, but their parents do not seem reassured. It is only when I discover that Great Aunt Mable had similar symptoms and she was crushed to death by a flock of stampeding hyenas and the parents worry if little Johnny's tummy noises might be mistaken as a hyena mating cry, that I can address what they are really worried about.
- Think about who you ask. You are clearly worried and anxious. If you ask everybody that you see what they think, then you will get a mix of different answers, which will confuse you. Try

to ask people who can give you the best answer. This can vary depending what you want to know. Whilst a consultant might have a good understanding about test results, the nursery nurse will undoubtedly know more about how your baby is feeding and handling and how to bathe him.

- Don't be fobbed off. It is not unreasonable for you to expect that the staff will keep you updated. However, clearly there are times when this will not be possible, because they will be doing other things. Sometimes there are fixed times when staff meets parents, so try to find out when these are.
- Think about who should be present. Whilst in an ideal world, medical staff would have limitless time to talk to everybody; the real world does not work like this. One of the frustrations is when I speak to a father for half an hour and then ten minutes later he approaches me and says "do you mind telling my wife what you just told me?"

In general, hospitals will only give information about babies to people with parental responsibility for them. This is for a number of reasons.

- He is your baby. You can tell your friends and family whatever you want and just because he is in hospital does not mean that they need to know all your secrets. You do not have to tell everybody everything and you may wish to keep some things private.
- We don't know who you don't get on with. There may be friends and family that you want nothing to do with. It is not our job to get involved in family arguments.
- We do also have to look after babies and we can't spend all day on the phone to everybody that has ever spoken to you, giving them updates.

So, in general, parents will receive information and everybody else will be asked to speak to them.

SCBU /NICU /NNU what's it to you?

Every delivery suite will have some facility for looking after babies who need extra care. These baby units use lots of different names such as SCBU (Special Care Baby Unit) NNU (Neonatal Unit) or NICU (Neonatal Intensive Care Unit) they might divide themselves further into rooms where babies need a lot of medical care (ITU - the Intensive Therapy Unit, ICU Intensive Care unit or Hot Rooms) a little less care (HDU - High Dependency Unit or warm rooms) or mainly nursing care (Nurseries or cold rooms).

Each unit will have staff and equipment to deal with a certain number of babies with different degrees of medical need. For example not every hospital will be able to manage very sick or extremely premature babies who will need to go to specialised units.

As much as possible, we try to make sure that your baby will deliver in a safe environment. If we know in advance that they will need a high level of care, your obstetric team will try and arrange that you deliver in a hospital that has the proper facilities for your baby. If you deliver somewhere else, your baby can be transferred to an appropriate environment, but this is less desirable.

Unfortunately, finding a suitable hospital for your baby is not always straightforward and whilst we try and find one as close as possible, there can be some travelling involved. Sometimes, you may be transferred to another hospital, but if things settle down and your baby seems safer you can be transferred back to deliver more locally.

Sometimes although your local unit may, in theory be able to look after your baby, they may be full. This means that they would be overstretched and not be able to provide a proper level of care. In these situations you may also be transferred to another hospital.

In situations where you have been transferred, everybody will do their best to get you to your local hospital as soon as it is safe to do so.

Being a SCBU Parent

Having a baby admitted to SCBU is often a very scary experience. The chances are that something unexpected has happened. Something has probably gone wrong and you have to face the fact that although we like to think that we have control over our lives, in reality, we actually have very little.

A lot of your anxiety is likely to be misplaced, as most SCBU admissions are for short term problems, but nevertheless, it can be disturbing to see your baby 'taken away' and being subjected to various things which although necessary are hardly pleasant.

Also, because you may not know what is going on, you can feel disempowered. If you touch your baby, will that make him sicker or interfere with his treatment? It can easily feel as if your baby is not really yours and you need to ask the SCBU team permission for everything: Can we take him out for a cuddle? Feed him? Change his nappy?

There will often be other parents around so you can't put on your funny voices. I think in all my years I have only heard one parent sing to their baby on a neonatal unit in a voice any louder than a whisper.

Although doctors and nurses realise that they do not own the babies on the unit, we sometimes can behave as if we do. It is important that you are the parents. Don't be afraid to ask for things that you want to happen or challenge those that you don't.

There are many communication difficulties, the most common one will be the simple 'absence of communication'. You may want to do something - such as dress or feed your baby and will wait for the nurses to give you 'permission' to do so. At the same time the nurses will be doing what you wanted to do, because you haven't so far shown any interest in doing it yourself! Because mindreading is only a desirable but not an essential attribute in our job description, it is hard for us to know what you want to do unless you tell us.

Many of the rules of a unit are, like most rules in life, fairly arbitrary. If you want to be able to do something and are told 'no', without being given a good reason, do not be afraid to challenge this and ask one of the senior members of the team.

Incubators and equipment

If you are unfamiliar with a neonatal unit, it can seem like a science fiction nightmare, with lots of machines making strange noises. Most of these are just there to keep things under control, simply to monitor your baby's situation and are not a sign of anything terrible going on.

There are numerous variations on the basic machines, each with varying amounts of bells and whistles, not forgetting the alarms. In fact, the identifying noise of the neonatal unit is usually the alarm. Each machine has one and any tiny change is likely to trigger it off. For example a baby might wriggle a bit and the monitor might become loose which will trigger the alarm to go off. Or a baby might have some trapped wind and catch their breath; again alarms will go off by the dozen. One of the skills of the neonatal team is knowing which alarms are actually important.

Let's take a walk through an average neonatal unit. First going to the place where the sickest babies are. Imagine looking into the room. You will hear some humming of machinery, a lot of alarms and some conversation. As you look in you will see a number of babies. They will either be in incubators or on small beds under heaters. Some of them will be under a strange blue light. The babies might need help breathing and will have a tube coming out of their mouths or nose, attached to some form of 'breathing machine'.

They will also be covered with sticky probes which lead off to a television like display, which shows lots of graphs and numbers. There are likely to be lots of drugs in syringes or bags going in through drips either through the baby's umbilical cord or through a drip in the hand or foot. So far all of this is normal, but it is worth just explaining what is happening.

How babies are managed varies in different hospitals. It is essential to ensure that they are kept warm and can be observed to receive all necessary care. The smaller the baby the more difficult it is to prevent them getting too cold. Very premature babies can also lose a lot of water through their skin so need to be kept in a very humid environment.

The best way to achieve all of this is to use some form of incubator. This allows us to keep a baby warm, but also allows us to monitor them closely and see them all the time. Sometimes it is important to be able to get near to the baby - for example to put in monitoring lines. It may be easier to have the baby on an open 'bed' with an overhead heater.

As babies become bigger and better at maintaining their own temperatures, they would normally be moved into a cot or bassinette. This is usually nothing much more than a plastic box. Being in an incubator is more often a sign of a baby's size rather than anything else.

Close by the incubator will be the monitoring equipment, which is usually displayed on a single television type screen. This will display graphs, numbers and 'squiggly lines'. These will be showing various measurements. Let's go through the things that we can often measure. Obviously how intensively a baby is monitored will depend on what exact needs they have.

- Temperature - There will often be a temperature probe attached to the baby's tummy. These are usually small round 'tin foil' looking probes. A normal temperature would be around 37 C
- Pulse (P) or Heart Rate (HR) which are effectively the same thing. There will usually be an ECG tracing next to this on the screen. The Normal level is usually around 120-160 beats per minute. Depending on other conditions, the team will only get concerned if the heart rate is less than 100 or more than 200. The ECG is measured via 3 small stickers which are placed on the baby.
- Respiratory Rate (R or Resp). This would usually be between 40 - 60 breaths per minute, but can vary greatly. If a baby is on a ventilator, it may be much slower and some conditions can mean that it is much higher. In general breathing at a rate less than 30 breaths per minute or more than 80 would need consideration. The ECG stickers and/or a ventilator can measure the respiratory rate.
- Blood Pressure (BP) this can be measured in one of two ways. Either by a normal - albeit baby sized - blood pressure cuff which is placed around the baby's arm or leg, or if the baby has an arterial line it can be measured through this with a special probe. There are two parts to the blood pressure the systolic, when the heart is pumping and the diastolic when the heart is 'filling up'. Blood pressure is usually measured in 'millimetres of mercury' (mmHg). In an adult the systolic blood pressure may be 110 and the diastolic 70, which would be written as 110/70. Children's blood pressures are usually much lower than adults. As well as the systolic and diastolic blood pressures, we also calculate the average or mean blood pressure (MBP). In general, with ill or premature babies we are more concerned by low rather than by high blood pressure. As a rule of thumb we like to keep the 'mean blood pressure' at the same as the gestation of the baby. So a 32 week baby should have a mean blood pressure above 32mmHG.
- Saturations (SaO2) Is a measure of how much 'oxygen is in the blood'. Normally this would be above 97% but, in some instances it is overall better to keep it a little lower. A much lower level of

saturations is not particularly dangerous of itself, but it does give us an idea of how severe a problem is. In some babies with heart abnormalities where the blood bypasses the lungs, the saturations may be as low as 70% and still not significantly affect the baby. A 'saturation probe' is usually a small piece of plastic which has a red light inside. It is wrapped around a finger or toe in bigger babies, or sometimes placed on an earlobe. In smaller babies it is usually wrapped around a wrist or ankle.

- Carbon Dioxide (CO_2) in babies who are being ventilated, or who have ongoing breathing problems, it is useful to know how much carbon dioxide is in the blood. We want to make sure it does not get too low, as this can then affect the blood supply to the brain, or get too high, as this is often a sign that the baby is not breathing properly. The most accurate way of measuring this is with a blood test, but it is also possible to measure the carbon dioxide through the skin, or if a baby is ventilated by measuring the carbon dioxide that is breathed out. Both of these methods give us an idea of what the baby's carbon dioxide levels are, but as they do not measure it directly, can not be used alone without checking the blood levels as necessary. In a baby with an arterial line, it is possible to make more or less continuous measurement of the levels in the blood. This is not used commonly for a number of reasons.

'Tubes going in and tubes coming out tubes everywhere'

Another inevitability of neonatal care is a number of tubes. Again it is probably most useful to go through these in turn. Not every baby will need everything; it depends on how premature or sick they are.

- Intravenous Cannulae or 'drips'. Most babies in neonatal care will at some stage need a cannula. This is a tube which goes into a vein to allow us to give drugs and fluids directly into the vein. If a baby needs a lot of intravenous drugs, they may need more than one cannula. The cannula is a little plastic tube. There is a needle inside the tube which is used to put the tube in place, but is then removed, so that it is only the plastic that stays in the vein. Usually the cannula will be covered with some form of bandage to ensure that it does not fall out or get pulled out.

- Long Lines. If babies can not feed for a short time, they can be given fluid intravenously (through a cannula into a vein). This will provide them with fluid, salt and sugar, but is only suitable for a short while, until proper feeding can be established. This is because the fluids do not provide a baby's entire requirement. So, babies who need prolonged intravenous feeding can receive a mixture known as 'Parenteral Nutrition' which does essentially provide them with a 'balanced diet'. However, Parenteral Nutrition does carry some minor risks, so we do not use it unless it is deemed necessary. One of the drawbacks of Parenteral Nutrition is that it can irritate the veins. In order to overcome this, it can be delivered via a 'long line'. This is a thin plastic tube which is inserted into a vein and then threaded up, until the tip is positioned in a big vein close to the heart. Placing 'long lines' can be quite intricate. Once in place, the part of the line outside the baby will be covered in sterile dressing and may be bandaged as well.
- Umbilical Lines: The umbilicus (belly button) provides us with fantastic access to a baby's veins and arteries. The umbilical cord has blood vessels within it which, before birth connect the baby to the placenta. At birth, the cord is cut. It is possible to pass small tubes through the blood vessels in the cord, directly to some of the big blood vessels in the baby.
- The Umbilical cord normally has two arteries. By passing an Umbilical Artery catheter (UAC) we can have continuous and painless access to a baby's arterial blood system. This allows us to measure:
  - ◊ Blood pressure
  - ◊ Oxygen and Carbon dioxide blood levels (blood gasses)

It also means that we can take blood tests painlessly.

There is also an Umbilical vein. Placing a tube in this - an Umbilical Venous Catheter (UVC) means that we have an easy way of administering any fluid intravenously. This is especially useful if babies are quite sick and need a lot of fluid and/or if they have difficult veins and obtaining other forms of access are proving difficult.

- Nasogastric/orogastric tubes: These are tubes which connect to the stomach, either through the nose (nasogastric) or mouth (orogastric). The two main reasons for these tubes are:

◊ Putting things into the stomach: such as milk and medications. As many premature babies are not able to suck and swallow properly, they will need to be fed through a tube until their own feeding skills develop.

◊ Taking things out of the stomach. Usually either air or gastric contents. If babies are swallowing lots of air, their stomachs can get distended and this can press on their lungs and make breathing more difficult. Also, in some babies who become sick, they stop being able to absorb feeds or even their own secretions and these may need to be 'sucked out'.

• Catheters: In some babies it is important to measure their urine production. In order to do this they may have a catheter placed in the bladder. In boys this will be through the penis and in girls through the vagina.

• Breathing tubes: Many babies, particularly those born prematurely will need help with breathing. This can be accomplished in many ways.

◊ Ventilator tubes (Endo Tracheal or ET tubes). These are used for babies on proper ventilators. A thick tube is passed through the mouth or nose into the windpipe (trachea). The tube is connected to the ventilator tubing.

◊ CPAP masks or prongs: CPAP (Continuous positive airways Pressure) is used in babies who need some help breathing, but not quite as much as a 'proper' ventilator. Basically air or oxygen is provided under pressure. To help keep the pressure a tight seal is needed around the baby's nose. This can be provided by a small triangular nose mask or with some nasal prongs. Both of these are held in place by some tight strapping around the baby's head.

◊ Nasal prongs. In babies who just need a little bit of oxygen, this can be delivered by nasal prongs. Here, a small ring of plastic piping which goes around the baby's head has two little protrusions which go into the nostrils. The oxygen is provided through the piping.

The other common feature of a neonatal unit is the lights used to combat jaundice. These can take the form of overhead lights or blankets which are placed under the baby. They emit a special UV glow which often provides the nursery with a characteristic appearance.

The equipment and monitoring highlighted above is used more or less routinely in every neonatal unit. If your baby does need to be admitted, then the staff should explain to you what everything is. It is important to remember that the majority of neonatal unit activity is about keeping things normal. Neonatologists are really just 'artificial placentas'. We do our best, but we do depend on a lot of monitoring.

Who gets admitted?

In most places in the UK about 1 in 10 babies will have some experience of needing some neonatal care. This means that the overwhelming majority will have no problems whatsoever.

Every hospital has a different setup. Some hospitals will admit most of these babies to their neonatal unit. Other hospitals have 'transitional care units' which look after babies who need only a small amount of help - for example they are a little premature and need to be kept warm or need a bit of help with feeding. In most cases the major difference is that in a transitional care unit, the mother or even both parents can stay with the baby, but in neonatal units this is usually not possible.

Babies may also receive treatment on the routine postnatal ward or paediatric wards. This depends on the level of treatment required and sometimes even just simple bed availability. When thinking about babies who are admitted to the neonatal unit, it is helpful to distinguish between those born prematurely and those born at full term. Let's talk about the full term babies first.

The most common reasons for admission are as follows:

- Too big or too small
- Poor feeding
- Cold - 'hypothermic'
- Low Blood sugar - 'hypoglycaemic'
- Signs of infection - 'sepsis'

- Jaundice
- Difficulty breathing - 'transient tachypnoea of the newborn'

Much less common, but more serious problems are:

- Birth Asphyxia - 'Hypoxic Ischaemic Encephalopathy'
- Meconium Aspiration
- Persistent Foetal Circulation /Persistent Pulmonary Hypertension of the Newborn
- Previously undiscovered abnormalities e.g. cardiac, genetic, surgical

Remember to keep things in context. The serious problems are rare, happening much less than 1 in 100 births. This is a great tribute to advances in maternity care and our great grandmothers would marvel at how much safer motherhood has become in the last few generations. So whilst there are still some improvements to be made, we can be quite proud of where we are. What we really need to do now is to export this safety around the world, so that every woman everywhere can expect that childbirth will be safe for her and her children.

Let's go through the lists and explain a few things.

Too big or too small:

Babies born too big or too small can have a number of issues. If they are born with a very high birth weight - the definition varies, but often will be around 4-4.5kg (9-10lbs) - then they are more likely to have problems with low blood sugar levels. They are also more likely to have had difficult deliveries so may have some birth trauma and bruising which can make jaundice worse.

Because doctors like using abbreviations, there are numerous medical names given for babies that are born too small; LBW Low Birth Weight, VLBW Very Low Birth Weight, SGA - Small for gestational age, SFD Small for dates.

Every small baby may have difficulty keeping themselves warm, but other problems depend on why a baby has been born small. Most babies that are born too small are just normal small babies and do not have other problems.

Some babies are born small because they have been 'underfed' in the womb. This normally occurs if the placenta has not been working as well as it should, it can happen if the mother has very high blood pressure or smokes, but often happens without any good reason. If the placenta cannot provide adequate nutrition for the baby then they will not grow properly.

In this situation, the placenta will be delivering less oxygen than expected. In order to deal with this the baby will make extra red blood cells (polycythaemia) to try and extract as much oxygen from the placenta as possible a consequence of this is that it causes the blood to 'thicken' and become sluggish.

These babies can have issues with falling blood sugars, because red blood cells consume a lot of glucose and if they are born too small they may have only limited energy stores in their body.

Another problem with polycythaemia is that it can reduce overall blood flow - because the blood is thicker and more sluggish. For example, this can have an impact on the bowel. In extreme cases, the blood reaching the bowel may be just enough to keep it alive whilst it is resting, but not enough if it has to start work at digesting milk. In this situation, it is often better to delay milk feeds or to start feeding slowly.

Because they can be 'fragile', very small babies are often safest being monitored for a few days.

Once they start feeding, we expect them to catch up and grow appropriately.

A very small group of small babies may have medical problems such as a genetic disorder or infection which have delayed growth. In this situation, they will need some investigations before considering proper management.

Poor Feeding/ Cold/ Low Blood Sugar:

These three often come together and one causes the other in a vicious cycle. After birth a baby may be a bit slow to feed, for example if the delivery has been difficult or if the mother has had some drugs during delivery. Or, if the room that they are in is cold they may become cold. Normally all

116

they require is warming up and feeding. Sometimes if they can not feed well, they may need feeding via a tube or a 'drip'. Because these symptoms can indicate an infection, some babies with these symptoms will receive antibiotics as well. Things usually get better quite quickly, over a day or so.

In some babies, particularly if the mother has had diabetes or poor glucose control (see above), the blood sugar difficulties may last a little longer.

Signs of infection - 'sepsis':

As we have mentioned before, most neonatologists are almost phobic about infection. 'If a baby cries they might be brewing something and if he doesn't cry it's probably even worse'. As a consequence any minor change in a baby is likely to trigger a response of treating with intravenous antibiotics. The reason for this is that infections can become very serious very quickly, so there is a tendency to excessive caution.

There is some suggestion that a more reasoned approach might be on the horizon, but essentially at present its still 'antibiotics all round'. Most times these will be given for somewhere between 2 and 5 days.

As most of these babies are treated 'just in case' it is not surprising that they do very well and we would not expect any long term problems. A tiny minority of children will have more significant signs of infection and they would require more attention than simply receiving antibiotics.

Jaundice:

As mentioned before, this is common. For most jaundiced babies no treatment is required. For many any treatment can usually be given on the postnatal ward. A few babies will have very high levels, or may need blood transfusions as well; this tiny number will usually be on the neonatal unit.

Difficulty breathing - 'transient tachypnoea of the newborn':

Before delivery, babies lungs are filled with lung liquid, which is resorbed before birth, so that at delivery, the lungs can fill with air. In some babies this does not happen quickly enough and at birth there is still some fluid in the lungs which makes breathing difficult. The liquid normally gets resorbed over the next day or so, but they may need help breathing during this time. Babies born by elective Ceasarean section, especially if done a few weeks before term are at a slightly higher risk of this occurring. They should recovery completely, with no long term problems.

Birth Asphyxia - 'Hypoxic Ischaemic Encephalopathy' (HIE):

This is what everybody dreads. It does only happen in about 1 in 1000 births so it is rare and there have been recent advances which have improved the outcome for babies. Essentially, this is when the baby is starved of oxygen and the lack of oxygen affects the brain and other organs.

This can lead to brain damage - specifically cerebral palsy. It used to be said that this was due to a difficult delivery and this is part of the reason why Caesarean Section rates have increased dramatically in the last 30 years. The idea being that if you avoid difficult delivery there would be no more children with cerebral palsy. Unfortunately, this has not proved to be the case, leading to the suggestion that the damage may have been caused some time before delivery and a baby with problems may have difficulty navigating the birth canal. So that more than difficult deliveries causing cerebral palsy, cerebral palsy causes difficult deliveries.

Babies with HIE are divided into three categories called the Sarnat Classification after the husband and wife team that described it. Type 1 is mild, type 2 is moderate and type 3 is severe, depending on their symptoms. Babies with Type 1 HIE are usually pretty well and may be just very irritable whereas at the other end babies with the most severe form may not be able to breathe for themselves or maintain their blood pressure, they may have fits and need a lot of intensive care.

Recently, it has been shown that cooling a baby with HIE can improve their outcome and this is becoming more widely available.

It is always difficult to know what the outcome is for a particular baby. Most babies with Type 1 HIE will have no problems at all, whereas in the Group with Type 3, it is unlikely that they will escape completely unscathed. Type 2 are somewhere in the middle.

Increasingly, special MRI scans can suggest what the degree of any damage is likely to be. Obviously, they are not 100% reliable and these scans are not widely available as yet.

Parents in this horrible situation will often want to know about the benefits of continuing care. This is such a personal discussion, that it can't be done justice in a book like this, but it is important to get as much information as is possible. I hope that this is a decision that nobody will have to make.

Persistent Foetal Circulation (PFC) /Persistent Pulmonary Hypertension of the Newborn (PPHN):

Because a baby in the womb does not breathe air, their circulation is organised so that only a small amount of blood goes through the lungs. After delivery, all of this has to change and all the blood has to flow through the lungs. Sometimes this change does not happen, for example if there is serious infection or meconium aspiration (see below). If the baby's circulation does not change then the blood will not be able to pick up oxygen, which is obviously very dangerous.

This is often a critical condition. Invariably babies with this condition will need to be on a ventilator and managing this can be very difficult. They will be treated with a number of drugs that alter the blood pressure in the lungs and body, as well as trying to treat any underlying cause. Occasionally babies will need a special treatment ECMO - which is effectively a lung bypass treatment. This is only carried out in a few centres in the UK.

Often during the first week it is 'touch and go'. After this stage, the situation usually improves and the circulation changes as it should have done in the first place. So, normally, if the first week has been overcome, there is very good recovery although it can take a long time.

Meconium Aspiration Syndrome (MAS):

Meconium is the first 'poo' that babies pass. If they are distressed before delivery they may pass this whilst still inside the womb. This means that the meconium gets into the amniotic fluid. Because distress can lead to gasping, the baby may then 'breathe in' this meconium stained fluid.

Because of this, if it is clear that a baby has passed meconium before delivery, then the midwives will make sure that plans are made for delivery. This might include sucking out the baby's mouth as soon as the head is delivered to make sure the baby is not going to breathe in a mouthful of meconium with his first breath. The baby may also be checked by a Paediatrician at birth. It is not clear if this makes much of a difference, as in most cases of meconium aspiration, the damage has occurred before delivery.

Although many babies will pass meconium before birth only a very small number will have meconium aspiration syndrome.

If meconium gets into the lungs it can cause a nasty chemical reaction which can seriously affect lung function. It can also trigger PFC/PPHN (see above). Babies with meconium aspiration syndrome can be very sick. The condition can take a week or so before any improvement is seen. Again although recovery may be slow, it should be complete, unless there have been any complications.

Previously undiscovered abnormalities e.g. cardiac, genetic and surgical:

As ultrasound skills and technology improve all the time, more and more problems are identified before delivery. It is amazing to think that only 40 years ago women might only find out that they were carrying twins at the time the second one delivered! But, the technology is not 100% and occasionally there are some problems that have not been picked up before delivery.

This would include some heart abnormalities and some genetic problems. Also included would be problems that would not be able to be detected before delivery. For example a baby who has a problem digesting milk would not be identified until they started drinking milk after birth.

In these situations, the treatment and outcome obviously depends on what exactly the problem is.

Prematurity:

The term premature covers a very wide group of babies with very different problems and outcomes. Technically a baby is considered premature or preterm if they are born at less than 37 completed weeks of gestation. In order to think about prematurity sensibly it is often divided into different categories:

Moderately preterm: born between 35 and 37 weeks
Very preterm: born between 29 and 34 weeks
Extremely preterm: born between 24 and 28 weeks

The main questions that every parent wants to know are 'what is the outlook for a premature baby?' and 'what problems will they have?' Before trying to answer these questions in general there are a few things that need to be considered.

- How premature are they: Obviously, the more premature, the more vulnerable a baby is. Life is a genuine miracle and it is mind-blowing how many things go on in the womb that are just right to produce a healthy baby. When babies are born prematurely, most of their systems are not properly developed and they are very fragile. Neonatologists do their best to try and provide everything that a baby would get from being inside the womb, but this can sometimes be too great a challenge - obviously the more premature a baby is, the more difficult they will be to manage.

- What caused the prematurity: If a baby is born prematurely, there is often a reason for this, such as an infection in the mother or baby, a medical problem with the mother or, trauma. Sometimes a baby will be delivered prematurely because the monitoring during pregnancy has identified that the baby is struggling in the womb, so is safest being delivered. For quite a number of premature babies we do not know what causes the prematurity. Clearly, the cause of the prematurity can determine how sick a baby may be and this can have an impact on how they fare after delivery.

Disability and Prematurity:

What is disability? Most people have their own ideas about how much treatment they want for themselves or their loved ones depending on what treatment is involved and what the patient is going to be like at the end of it and this would apply to babies too. It is not the purpose of this book to go into this in great depth other than to say that these are impossible decisions to make and we should not judge others until we have stood in their shoes.

It is clear that being a patient on an intensive care unit is no picnic and a neonatal intensive care unit is no different. However much we try to make it comfortable, we know that there is a lot of discomfort and painful procedures. Added to this, the burden of having a child in hospital for months can be great and although we say that we expect most babies to be discharged around the time that they are due to be born, for very premature babies, they may be in hospital for considerably longer. Some or all of this time may be in a hospital a long way from the family home.

If the outcome from all of this was a healthy baby, then most people would agree that it would be worthwhile. Unfortunately, in babies born extremely prematurely, or at the limits of viability this is often not the case. And to go through all of the difficulties of neonatal care in this case may seem less reasonable.

There are often a number of difficult decisions to make. Should treatment start, continue or be withdrawn. This decision can be made easier if there are obvious problems with the baby which will almost certainly cause long term issues; in many situations it is, unfortunately, not so clear cut.

When people study the long term outcome of premature babies, they often have some very strange views about what is considered a disability. For instance a squint or needing to wear glasses is often classed as a mild disability, when most people would just think it as more or less normal. This means that when people say there is a certain chance of being disabled, it is more important to know what they mean by disabled.

Being politically incorrect, a former teacher of mine felt that it would be better to categorise the disabilities as:

- More or less normal
- Minor problems that 'we can live with'
- Major problems

I think that this makes practical sense, but unfortunately does not seem to have caught on.

If you are in this horrible situation of having to make a choice it is important that you have as much information as you possibly can. Because the choices are so emotive, you may feel pressured by others including doctors and nurses to make a decision that you do not want to make.

You may need to be strong and whichever decision you make you may need support from family friends and often from support organisations or professionals such as s GP or psychologist.

About 8% of all babies are born prematurely, but most of these are only moderately preterm. Let's explore prematurity by increasing gestation.

Babies born at around 24 weeks of gestation - that is 4 months early - are said to be at the extremes of viability. Essentially their lungs are so immature that they are often unable to breathe properly, even on a ventilator. Because all of their systems are so poorly developed, they often get many complications. The most significant of these is brain damage.

Giving figures for survival at this age is complicated and the outlook improves with every day if not every hour, of gestation. Because managing these babies is highly specialised, babies that are born in units designed to deal with them, will do better than those that are born at other hospitals and need to be transferred after delivery. In general, obstetric teams will try to get ladies who are in premature labour to a place where their baby can have the best possible outcome. Sometimes, the transfer can be too dangerous to undertake before the baby is born.

Remarkably about 50% of all babies born at 22 weeks gestation can survive and this figure increases to about 80% of children born at 24 weeks. However, these children usually require prolonged intensive care and often have significant long term problems. The decision about whether to resuscitate babies at this age or to let nature take its course is always heart rending.

Remarkably as described, by 24 weeks gestation - that is 4 months early, over 80% of babies survive, with probably about half of these having significant problems. By 28 weeks, survival rates will be more than 90%, with the vast majority of survivors having no major problems. Babies born at over 30 weeks gestation - that is still 10 weeks early - should have essentially the same survival chances as a baby born at full term.

Most of the research on how premature babies are when they grow up, has focussed on the extremely premature babies. Recent work looking at babies born only slightly prematurely has raised questions as to whether they have more than their fair share of minor problems. It is quite hard to measure this and these are often the kind of problems that you would expect in children born at term. Up to date information about everything is available from www.marchofdimes.com

The increased survival of premature babies is one of the major advances of modern medicine. The fact that most survive without long term problems is amazing. Frequent advances mean that the survival figures are getting better all the time.

What problems do premature babies have?

The problems of a premature baby become less; the closer they are to term. So whilst a baby born at 24 weeks is likely to have most or all of the problems outlined below, a baby born at 34 weeks is likely to have no more problems than if he was born at term. The list includes some of the major problems that a premature baby and the neonatal unit have to deal with.

Brain:

During pregnancy and in the early years of life, the brain grows and develops at a phenomenal rate. Although a baby's brain can often recover from some damage (an attribute known as plasticity), it is still very vulnerable. Small changes to blood flow and oxygen levels can have profound changes on the brain. The other problems that very premature babies have make it hard to control their blood pressure and oxygen levels at all times, which makes them vulnerable to brain damage. Premature babies' blood vessels, in certain areas of the brain, are especially fragile. This makes it easier for them to bleed. This will normally be monitored by ultrasound scans. Minor bleeds are often of little long term significance, but more major bleeds obviously are. The risk of bleeding reduces dramatically with gestation, so it is rare after about 30 weeks of gestation and almost unheard of after 34 weeks.

Eyes:

Very premature babies are prone to a condition called 'retinopathy of prematurity'. This is caused by oxygen 'damaging' the eye. To try to prevent this, we try to give babies that need extra oxygen, as little as possible. Very premature babies will have their eyes checked every week or so. Again by 30 weeks the risk of developing retinopathy is minimal. Children who are affected can have long term visual problems.

Feeding:

Babies need to grow. Getting them to do so can be difficult. Ideally they are started on breast milk as soon as possible. However, if babies are sick, they may not be sending enough blood to their intestines, which makes feeding dangerous, so feeds will usually be started quite slowly and built up gradually. In the interim they will receive nutrition through their veins, either sugar water, or ideally TPN (see above) the decision of which to use depends on many factors. Most babies over 32 weeks of gestation will not need TPN and should be on milk feeds fairly quickly. Babies learn to suck and swallow at about 34-37 weeks of gestation. This means that before this age they are likely to need feeding through a tube. Again, once feeding is established it should proceed normally. However, some children who have been ventilated for a long time or who have been tube fed for longer than expected, may have difficulties feeding later. Premature babies are prone to suffering with gastro-oesophageal (acid) reflux and often need treatment for this. They should over time outgrow this. Once feeding is established, premature babies often need extra vitamins and iron, to help them grow and these are usually continued for quite a few months. There are special milk formulas that are available for premature babies. What is recommended will vary in different hospitals.

Lungs:

This is often the big one in neonatal units. Babies' lungs grow dramatically in the last few months of pregnancy. Before 24 weeks of gestation they will have very immature lungs, which may be too poorly developed to work. After this stage the lungs will start to develop in a way that is more compatible with breathing. One of the vital things that is produced is a chemical called surfactant. This helps to keep the lungs open. In the absence of surfactant the lungs will collapse easily, which makes breathing more difficult. Surfactant is usually present in adequate quantities by about 34 weeks of gestation. Babies born earlier are more likely to have surfactant deficiency. This presents in a typical way and is known as Respiratory Distress Syndrome (RDS) or Hyaline Membrane Disease (HMD). One of the major advances in neonatal care has been the use of animal surfactant to treat this condition. Babies who show signs of surfactant deficiency can be treated with this animal surfactant. It is extremely safe and usually brings about a dramatic improvement. It does not always solve the problem and they may still need help with breathing. Another massive advance has been the discovery that if mothers of premature babies are given steroids before delivery, their babies will have fewer breathing problems - there is still some uncertainty as to which the best steroid to use is and when and how often they should be given. Despite these advances making sure that a baby is breathing effectively can be a very great challenge. There are many different techniques for helping a baby breathe, depending on how much help they need. Although surfactant will usually be produced naturally by a baby after a few days of life, regardless of gestation, sometimes the damage that has been caused before this can take a long time to heal. Some babies might need breathing support for a very long time.

The good news is that as babies grow, their lungs should get better and better. Even in the worst situations, after a few years they should be effectively normal. As with all of these problems, they are more severe the more premature the baby and babies born at 32 weeks gestation and above are likely to have no or only minor breathing issues.

Heart:

Babies hearts are normally formed, most of the heart develops in the first few months of pregnancy and from then on there will not be any new problems. Premature babies should not have any more long term heart problems than babies born at term. Because of the different requirements before and after birth, there are as we have mentioned before, a few connections which need to change after delivery. Sometimes this can be allowed to happen. Premature babies are more likely to have a 'Patent Arterial Duct' This is a blood vessel that connects the main blood vessel going to the body (aorta) with the one going to the lungs (Pulmonary Artery). In the womb this allows blood to bypass the lungs. After birth it should close over a few days. In premature babies it often stays open. This can cause a number of problems including placing extra pressure on the heart and lungs. Sometimes, it does not cause any major problem and can be left till the baby is older. If it is causing problems, then it might close in response to medication or may need a small operation. Premature babies, especially very premature babies, can also have problems with

126

blood pressure. Again this is a short term problem, but they may need to have drugs for a short time to help maintain a normal blood pressure.

Jaundice:

Premature babies are probably more prone to jaundice because their livers are more immature and cannot 'process' the jaundice as well. They are also more prone to bruising which will make jaundice worse. Also, if they are being fed intravenously, the 'food' can sometimes make the jaundice worse. Probably more importantly is the fact that they are more vulnerable to the effects of jaundice, so a level that would be considered safe in a term baby may be considered dangerous in a premature baby. As long as the jaundice level is kept from rising too high, there should be no long term consequences.

Kidneys, Fluid and Sugar balance:

These are major challenges for neonatologists - ensuring that a baby gets neither dehydrated nor waterlogged. There are a number of factors which make this difficult. For example very premature babies may lose a lot of water through their skin and may need a lot of fluid to stop them dehydrating. As the fluids will usually contain sugar, they could risk having sugar levels that are too high.

Alternatively, in other situations, they may be producing very little urine. In this case, because the only way of giving them glucose is with fluid, it can be hard to give them enough glucose without overfilling them with water.

Often the only way to assess this is by frequent blood tests and weighing. Again these are problems essentially of the very premature baby and do not continue in the long term.

Skin:

Because premature babies' skin is quite thin, they are prone to bruising and getting pressure sores. It is also easier for things to travel though the skin, whether this is water getting out or infections getting in. In order to limit the water (and heat) loss through the skin, babies are usually placed in incubators which are kept at a fairly high temperature and with a high humidity. As they mature their skin will become normal.

Infection:

Premature babies are very prone to infections. They have an immature immune system and have missed the major transfer of protective antibodies that cross the placenta in the last few months of pregnancy. They have fragile skin and usually lots of lines and tubes in their bodies. Infection in these babies can be rapidly serious. Because of this, in most units, whenever a baby does anything untoward the neonatologists will worry about an infection and start antibiotics

Growth:

Growth is essential. It is the only way a baby can escape the neonatal unit. This can be difficult to achieve at the beginning - as the calorie requirements might be quite high and with a limited amount of fluid allowed every day, much of it could be taken up with drugs leaving little left over for food.

Once a baby does start growing this should continue normally and there should be no long term growth problems which are linked to being premature.

Taking your baby home:

Leaving SCBU can often be as hard if not harder as having to go there in the first place. It is easy to become reliant on the technology and the nurses to know that everything is alright. You will have spent so many hours looking at monitors and using them to reassure you that your baby is OK that it can be hard living without them. Most neonatal units will have the facility to allow you to spend some time on the unit, in a side room. So called 'rooming in'. This is aimed at trying to let you gain some confidence in looking after your baby by yourself.

When you finally get home and close the front door, the fact that you are on your own now, can trigger quite a bit of anxiety. You will probably spend the first few days and nights checking on your baby every few minutes. Usually this settles down quite quickly, normally due to exhaustion. If you find that you are becoming increasingly anxious, then you should discuss this with your GP, Health Visitor or midwife.

Stillbirth/Neonatal Death

Whilst I would love to bury my head in the sand and ignore these distressing topics, I think that we do need to mention them. Advances in medical care have made these rare events, but they are still tragic. Often no cause is ever found for this disaster, which is attributed to being 'just one of those things'. Sometimes there is a reason, which may be that somebody made a mistake. I don't know which situation is worse. All of this happens at a time when it is hard to grasp exactly what is going on. Most people do not know what to say or how to deal with a grieving family and this can include healthcare professionals.

In general I think it is important to acknowledge the existence of the baby. Who has been a part of the family's life and will always be there. It is comforting to know that 'you will never get over him'. Whenever possible I try to ensure that as much evidence of a baby's life, however brief, is recorded.

The legal system in the UK does not often take into account people's feelings and in the case of a stillborn baby, will not register the baby. Wherever possible I try to arrange the baby to have the facility to have a birth and death certificate. It is important to spend time with the baby and take as many pictures as needed. Older siblings are often encouraged to see the baby. You can't pretend it never happened and what they imagine is often worse than the reality. Getting back from this disaster is always hard. There are many bereavement organisations including SANDS the Stillbirth and Neonatal Death Society www.uk-sands.org

One of the most difficult things for grieving parents is the reaction of people around them. Many people do not know what to say. I have heard of friends crossing the other side of the street to avoid talking to a grieving couple and also of many comments that are so ludicrously insensitive that you wonder how any person could make them. Most people are probably well meaning but they just don't know how to show it properly.

In my experience, the last thing you want people to do is to minimize the tragedy. You will never get over it. And even if 'you can always have another one' (pretty high on the list of insensitive comments) the idea that somehow that replaces the lost baby is really quite offensive.

If you are pregnant after having experienced this loss, you are likely to need extra help during and after any future pregnancies and most hospitals should have some way of dealing with this.

I hope that you have found some or all of this book helpful and reassuring. My hope was that it would make you less worried about pregnancy and delivery. If I have made you more worried then I apologise. If you think that there are things that I have missed or should not talk about, or if you have any ideas then please let me know. I cannot answer specific questions but would value your comments.

I hope that everything goes well and you bring each other much joy

Anthony Cohn

anthony@anthonycohnpaediatrics.co.uk

CPSIA information can be obtained
at www.ICGtesting.com
Printed in the USA
LVHW082304020620
657270LV00014B/340

9 781908 586582